Dr Clare Grace is a regist......
ised in managing weight a.......................
worked in two specialist NHS clinics for people managing severe and complex obesity. She is currently a member of the Community Diabetes team at Leeds Community Healthcare Trust.

She has published a number of academic papers on issues relating to the management of weight and is a member of the British Dietetic Association (BDA), the BDA Obesity specialist group, the Association for the Study of Obesity, and is a member of the education committee of SCOPE, an international obesity training and certification programme for health professionals.

Dr Vicky Lawson is Principal Health Psychologist at Talking Therapies Southwark, London, and the Psychology Clinical Champion for Physical Activity for Public Health England. Vicky has worked for over fifteen years as a clinician, researcher and public health consultant, investigating how behaviour change strategies and the implementation of psychological methods can help to unpick the complexity of why we can struggle to make lifestyle changes. She has published widely on health psychology in a range of journals. She is a member of the British Psychological Society and the Health and Care Professions Council.

Dr Jeremy Gauntlett-Gilbert is a Clinical Psychologist who focuses on helping people with chronic physical health problems; he has worked at specialist NHS services for people with obesity, and currently specialises in the treatment of chronic pain.

Dr Gauntlett-Gilbert is a member of both the British Psychological Society and the British Association for Behavioural and Cognitive Psychotherapies (BABCP).

The aim of the **Overcoming** series is to enable people with a range of common problems and disorders to take control of their own recovery programme.

Each title, with its specially tailored programme, is devised by a practising clinician using the latest techniques of cognitive behavioural therapy – techniques which have been shown to be highly effective in changing the way patients think about themselves and their problems.

Many books in the Overcoming series are recommended under the Reading Well scheme.

Titles in the series include:

OVERCOMING ALCOHOL MISUSE, 2ND EDITION
OVERCOMING ANGER AND IRRITABILITY, 2ND EDITION
OVERCOMING ANOREXIA NERVOSA, 2ND EDITION
OVERCOMING ANXIETY, 2ND EDITION
OVERCOMING BODY IMAGE PROBLEMS INCLUDING BODY
DYSMORPHIC DISORDER
OVERCOMING BULIMIA NERVOSA AND
BINGE-EATING, 3RD EDITION
OVERCOMING CHILDHOOD TRAUMA
OVERCOMING CHRONIC FATIGUE, 2ND EDITION
OVERCOMING CHRONIC PAIN, 2ND EDITION
OVERCOMING DEPERSONALISATION AND
FEELINGS OF UNREALITY, 2ND EDITION
OVERCOMING DEPRESSION, 3RD EDITION
OVERCOMING DISTRESSING VOICES, 2ND EDITION
OVERCOMING GAMBLING ADDICTION, 2ND EDITION
OVERCOMING GRIEF, 2ND EDITION
OVERCOMING HEALTH ANXIETY
OVERCOMING HOARDING
OVERCOMING INSOMNIA AND SLEEP PROBLEMS
OVERCOMING LOW SELF-ESTEEM, 2ND EDITION
OVERCOMING MILD TRAUMATIC BRAIN INJURY AND
POST-CONCUSSION SYMPTOMS
OVERCOMING MOOD SWINGS
OVERCOMING OBSESSIVE COMPULSIVE DISORDER
OVERCOMING PANIC, 2ND EDITION
OVERCOMING PARANOID AND
SUSPICIOUS THOUGHTS, 2ND EDITION
OVERCOMING PERFECTIONISM, 2ND EDITION
OVERCOMING RELATIONSHIP PROBLEMS, 2ND EDITION
OVERCOMING SEXUAL PROBLEMS, 2ND EDITION
OVERCOMING SOCIAL ANXIETY AND SHYNESS, 2ND EDITION
OVERCOMING STRESS
OVERCOMING TRAUMATIC STRESS, 2ND EDITION
OVERCOMING WEIGHT PROBLEMS
OVERCOMING WORRY AND GENERALISED ANXIETY
DISORDER, 2ND EDITION
OVERCOMING YOUR CHILD'S SHYNESS AND SOCIAL ANXIETY
STOP SMOKING NOW, 2ND EDITION

OVERCOMING WEIGHT PROBLEMS

2nd Edition

*A self-help guide using
cognitive behavioural techniques*

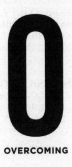

OVERCOMING

DR CLARE GRACE, DR VICKY LAWSON AND
DR JEREMY GAUNTLETT-GILBERT

ROBINSON

ROBINSON

First published in Great Britain in 2019 by Robinson

Copyright © Dr Clare Grace, Dr Vicky Lawson and
Dr Jeremy Gauntlett-Gilbert, 2019

Previous edition *Overcoming Weight Problems* written by Dr Clare Grace and
Dr Jeremy Gauntlett-Gilbert and published by Robinson,
an imprint of Constable & Robinson Ltd., 2005

1 3 5 7 9 10 8 6 4 2

A CIP catalogue record for this book
is available from the British Library.

IMPORTANT NOTE
This book is not intended as a substitute for medical advice or treatment.
Any person with a condition requiring medical attention should consult a
qualified medical practitioner or suitable therapist.

ISBN: 978-1-47214-288-7

Typeset in Bembo by Initial Typesetting Services, Edinburgh
Printed and bound in Great Britain by Clays Ltd, Elcograf S.p.A.

Papers used by Robinson are from well-managed forests and
other responsible sources.

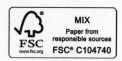

Robinson
An imprint of
Little, Brown Book Group
Carmelite House
50 Victoria Embankment
London EC4Y 0DZ

An Hachette UK Company
www.hachette.co.uk
www.littlebrown.co.uk

Contents

Introduction   1

PART ONE:
The Foundations

1   Motivation to change   31

2   Thoughts and beliefs   58

3   Self-awareness   92

PART TWO:
Making Changes

4   Changing physical activity   127

5   Changing eating habits   162

6   Making the changes in daily life   212

7   Eating to manage emotions   247

8   Dealing with other people's reactions   283

9   Keeping it going   328

Appendix I – Planning and recording   359

Appendix II – Taking it further   375

Index   387

Acknowledgements

This book draws on clinical and academic experience from psychology and dietetics to present an approach to managing weight and health that we hope will guide people to find ways of improving their quality of life.

We are indebted to the many patients who over the years have trusted us with their stories of weight gain, how this has impacted on their lives, and the challenges of making and sustaining changes to eating and activity habits. It is this understanding of the lived experience that guides our practice and our continued endeavours to improve the care and support given to those who are trying to manage their weight and health in challenging times.

Over the years we have been fortunate to work with a number of colleagues who have inspired the way we practice and so have contributed to the ideas we have presented in this book, directly or indirectly. Most notably: Professor Jane Wardle and Dr Helen Croker; Weight Concern; the Talking Therapies Southwark team; Professor Peter Kopelman; Professor Carolyn Summerbell; Professor Trisha Greenhalgh; Dr Simon Aylwin and Dympna Pearson.

Introduction

Many people are committed to making changes to their weight, eating and activity for their health or for some other important personal reason. They may have tried many different diets over the years but none have worked in the long term.

This is interesting, isn't it? Most people with larger bodies have taken steps to try to reduce their weight. They have very sensibly looked around them and seen what is recommended as the best way to do it, and the answer comes back: 'Go on a diet.'

It is fair to say that lots of people are currently on diets! Across the world there must be millions of people trying to lose weight this way. And of course there are also many different types of diets and always someone telling us: 'This is the best way to do it.' An incredible amount of energy is being put into this, making some people an incredible amount of money. People have followed diets promising that particular foods are the 'magic cure', or even that foods are good or bad in particular combinations.

Is it working? Well, about a third of people across the world are overweight, so perhaps most of these 'cures' have not been a great success. Some quick-fix 'diets' do work for some people in the short term. We have heard stories of those who have lost 5 or 10 stone through dieting. However, as soon as the diet is 'broken', the weight goes back on. As NHS clinicians, we have seen people who have been overweight for years, and very often for decades. They have usually been through the 'yo-yo' pattern of regularly losing weight and putting it all (or more) back on, and they often feel hopeless about the situation.

Many people have had such bad experiences with 'dieting' they blame themselves. They think they must be particularly lazy or weak-willed to have such a problem with their weight. Or perhaps they decide that they must have particular psychological problems with food. However, we think that someone who has spent many years struggling with diets is far from lazy! Unfortunately, there are many people, including some health professionals, who think people with larger bodies just need to 'pull their socks up' and 'eat less and exercise more'. This is like a business consultant telling an ailing company, 'Well, you just need to sell more of your products. Then you'll make more money.' The advice is correct, of course, but without any details of *how you would do that*, it is useless.

Knowing *how* to do it – how to eat differently, how to be more active, in a way that fits with our lives – seems to be strangely absent from most of the information we are bombarded with about weight and eating. It's all very well being given a diet and exercise plan to follow but what happens when you are too busy to buy and cook all the new healthy

2

foods you need to eat? Or you don't like them? Or they're too expensive? Or they don't have them at your local shop? Or you want go out with friends? Or you just want to eat some chocolate and nothing else will do? Knowing *how* to respond to these and many other situations rarely makes it into the latest diet fad but this can really make a difference.

We have seen people successfully manage their weight through simple changes to their food intake and activity levels. For someone who has spent ten years losing weight through diets and then putting it back on, permanent weight loss like this is a huge achievement. And people *can* do it, even if they have been trying for years. We know this from our clinical experience and from scientific studies (more about this later).

We wrote this book because we believe many of the challenges in managing weight can be helped by altering the focus of change. This means having a better understanding of what you are doing now, knowing what motivates you, and having a clear plan of what you need to change, rather than someone else telling you what you need to change. We are a dietitian, a health psychologist and a clinical psychologist. Whilst we cannot give you all of our professional training, we will try to pass on some of our skills and knowledge, including all of the 'top tips' – the most useful information on managing weight for the long term. You can then apply this in combination with your own expertise about yourself to come up with an approach that is centred on what is most likely to work for you.

Before we get started, it's helpful to have a better understanding of some broader questions before moving on to the alternative approach:

- Why are so many people overweight?
- Why don't quick-fix 'diets' work in the long term?

Why are so many people overweight?

There has been a significant rise in the last few decades in the number of people who are overweight. Why is this happening? Has there been a sudden global increase in 'laziness' or 'lack of willpower' across the world? Or has something happened in society that is making it harder and harder to be a healthy weight? As you can probably already guess, the answer to this question isn't simple and experts have identified quite a few different factors involved. One thing many of us can agree on is that the availability, range and relative cheapness of less-healthy foods have exploded in recent years.

It's really easy to eat more than our bodies need

So, how has it become easier to eat more? Portion sizes have definitely changed: something called 'portion distortion'. Standard packets of food are becoming bigger and the average size of a meal is getting larger in many restaurants. The size of a portion of chips in fast-food restaurants is quietly getting bigger and bigger. Food manufacturers know

4

that people like a bargain. If a person sees '50% extra free', or 'buy one get one free', they are likely to think they have saved money. Even the size of the average dinner plate has increased by several inches.

The dangerous thing about 'portion distortion' is we *might not change our eating habits at all*, but the amount we eat would still go up. Here's an example of how dangerous this effect can be:

- In the 1980s, the average packet of crisps weighed 25g. These days single packets of crisps weigh just over 32g. Imagine a person who eats five packets of crisps a week. . .
- If they eat five of the 32g packets, that's the same as eating six and a half of the old 25g packets.
- So switching to the 32g bags is like eating one and a half extra bags per week.
- Or 6 bags per month.
- Or 75 bags extra per year!
- Over five years, this person would eat an extra 9.5kg of crisps without changing their eating habits at all.

Of course, most people don't just buy single packs – crisps either come in 'sharing' 100g-plus bags or multipacks of six, so there is even more opportunity to overeat. And it's not just crisps. If you look around you, 'portion distortion' is everywhere. A coffee-shop 'cookie' was once the size of a biscuit – these days it is likely to be the size of a small plate. Also, it's not always clear how much energy (calories) we are consuming: the combination of a large latte and a blueberry muffin contains about the same calories as a main meal. In addition, many foods that are marketed as being healthy are far from that for people who are trying to manage their weight.

This is only part of the story. If you take a trip through most cities, it is amazing to see how many shops sell fast food, fried food and takeaways. Think of the number of all-you-can-eat buffets, extra-huge pizzas and free offers. It's also obvious that these days there are many more exciting – and fattening – foods to enjoy. Think of the new ranges of ice-cream flavours or deep-fried crisps on offer. They often taste delicious and are marketed in a way that makes us want to try them. Unfortunately, it can be difficult to enjoy them in moderation. . . Food seems to have become a much bigger part of our lives, with a profusion of television shows, podcasts and magazine articles glamorising food and ensuring it is ever-present. Even *when* we are able to buy food has changed: in the UK, supermarkets weren't allowed to open on Sundays until 1994.

So we are definitely being tempted to eat more, and it is easier to do so, and not be aware that it is happening. This would be less of a problem if activity also increased to the same degree. But. . .

We are spending less time being active

Again, it's not the case that we have suddenly become lazy. It has just becoming easier and easier to sit still – we have engineered activity out of our lives, from cars to escalators to lifts, dishwashers and, of course, screens. We spend a large proportion of our time sitting in front of a screen in some form or other. Many parts of modern life that make us sit still are great. Films, TV shows, games and the internet can provide fantastic entertainment. We can do such an amazing number of things with a home computer. Mobile phones are incredibly useful and save lots of time. Where would we be without our cars and TVs? But the result is less activity. We don't even need to be active to get our food any more, with supermarket delivery services, and takeaways at the touch of a button; everything is available from our sofas.

So here is the picture: we live in an environment that tends to make it difficult for people to control their weight by persuading them to eat more and be less active. Alongside this, we have a human survival instinct hardwired into our brains to want to eat high-energy foods (those with lots of fat and sugar) and not move around too much. This is because for most of human existence food was extremely scarce and we needed to be active to find food or be able to produce it ourselves.

How we feel about our bodies, and other people's

Over-abundant food supply and easy options to avoid activity aren't the only problems. There are also the attitudes about what ideal bodies 'should', and 'shouldn't', look like – and much of this comes from how the media and fashion industries portray people. In films, for example, if someone is overweight, particularly if they are female, they are less likely to be taken seriously, to be the romantic lead or to be the action lead. And even if they are, it is usually thought necessary to comment on their body size.

And of course, while the media shapes our views it also reflects our attitudes. We live in a society where people are constantly comparing themselves to someone else and making judgements about other people based on what they look like. This has only increased (got worse!) since the rise of social media platforms like Instagram and Facebook. Thinness is promoted as an ideal whilst being overweight as the opposite. This has very real consequences for people who are overweight and research has shown those with larger bodies are often discriminated against, in jobs, healthcare, at school and in general day-to-day life. Negative attitudes based on weight are often seen as a totally acceptable form of discrimination, which of course they are not. It's an odd situation – we live in a society that encourages people to gain weight but then punishes those who do. On the other hand, slimness is portrayed as necessary for success and happiness. Pictures of very thin women or lean but muscly men are everywhere and there is a public obsession with which celebrities have lost – or put on – weight. The fashion industry generally tries to sell a body image that is impossible for the vast majority of the population to achieve and even the models in the pictures have usually been airbrushed.

We have colleagues who work with people with anorexia, a condition that is more likely to result in death than any other psychiatric disorder. Yet some fashion models clearly have a weight that is in the anorexic range. And they are meant to be a good example of beauty. In more recent years, there has been an increase in more curvy models, which is some progress, but 'curvy' is defined by some leading model agencies as women over a UK size 10 (USA size 8).

You may think we're exaggerating. However, we are very serious. Have a look at the dummies used to display women's clothes in shop windows. A study in the *British Medical Journal* showed if these shop dummies were real women, they would be so dangerously thin they would no longer be able to menstruate. Yet these are supposed to be the 'ideal shape' for women.

You may well be aware of these attitudes from your own experiences. However, less well known are the consequences for people who are trying to manage their weight. Sometimes people say, 'But surely some of these negative attitudes towards being overweight are a good thing? Don't they help motivate people to change?' The answer to this is no! If negative attitudes towards being overweight were helpful it would then follow that people would find it much easier to lose weight, which of course they do not. In fact the opposite is true. Research has shown that people who are discriminated against because of their body size are actually much *more* likely to overeat; food may be used as a comfort following an upsetting experience or it may be a way of rebelling – 'You can't tell me what to do.'

Why don't quick-fix 'diets' work in the long term?

So, if we are living in a world where we are encouraged to eat more than we need, where it is all too easy to be inactive, and where unhealthily thin body shapes are admired, then it's understandable that many people try to 'fix' their weight as quickly as they can.

Of course, the first thing to be said about quick-fix 'diets' is they can work – for a while. People who go on them often manage to lose a few pounds, and sometimes even more. If we only needed to change our eating habits in the short term, so we could look good for a special occasion, for example, then traditional quick-fix solutions might be fine.

Yet what so many people need more help with is how to keep weight off for the long term. In order to do this, we need to find an eating and activity plan that we can imagine doing for the rest of our lives. Who can imagine following some of the quick-fix 'diets' for the rest of their lives? This is the problem – and here are some reasons why:

They are not very flexible or interesting

Rigid 'diets' with very restrictive rules about what you 'should' and 'shouldn't' eat just don't fit with most people's lifestyles over the long term. They might be simple and easy to follow initially – you just have to eat what you are told. However, we were not designed to eat the same things every day. Most people go out for dinner once in a while, or have a takeaway. How does this fit with a strict set of rules? And how many of us would be willing to give up going out for dinner *for ever*?

They tell us to stop eating certain foods

Most of us know that as soon as we are told we 'can't' eat something, we begin to crave it and thoughts of it will pop into our head all of the time. Needless to say, this is not going to work well for managing weight. How many people would be willing to spend the rest of their lives without eating chocolate (or crisps or cheese)? Any diet that 'bans' foods and suggests there are 'good' and 'bad' foods isn't helpful.

They are designed to be short-term

This is the basic problem with most quick-fix 'diets'. Most sell the idea that you can do something *for a short period of time*, and then your weight problem will be fixed *for ever*. This will not happen. As soon as someone returns to their old eating and activity habits weight gain is likely to occur.

This promise of a short-term 'fix' can be seen in many areas of life. For example, for those with debt problems there are lots of adverts saying something like: 'Take out a big loan from us – you can pay off your credit cards and all of your other debts at once.' Of course, this is true. But if the person who takes the loan does not fix the basic problem – they are spending more than they earn – then no short-term 'fix' will help. It's just the same for managing weight – if a person does not change their regular eating and activity habits, no quick-fix solution will help. This leads us to another problem with many quick-fix solutions. . .

They ignore activity – or don't treat it as very important

Many approaches to managing weight focus mainly on food. This is a problem. Lots of recent scientific research shows activity is very important in preventing weight gain in the first place and in helping people keep weight off long-term. The other thing that recent research tells us is that people who are more active have much better mental and physical health overall. As you can imagine, this is going to be really helpful when it comes to making long-term changes to what we eat. So if we are thinking about weight management for the long term, we can't ignore activity.

They are often based on a 'fad' theory of how to manage weight

There are so many 'diets' that claim to have found the magical cure to permanent weight loss. 'If you just follow this special formula, your weight will disappear quickly and easily.' It would be wonderful if this were true. However, these 'diets' often have no good-quality scientific evidence to support their claims. It is better to put your time and effort into approaches more likely to be of help to you.

Of course, some people will lose weight by using the 'magical' approaches – however, this will have something to do with the overall change to their eating habits and nothing at all to do with the 'fad' theory behind it.

The bottom line

What is needed is to find a way of eating that you enjoy, that includes a good balance of healthy foods, gives you flexibility so favourite foods can be included, and fits into your routine and lifestyle. It's important to recognise that there isn't one perfect solution or one type of diet/approach for managing health and weight – rather there are a number of different eating patterns or diets which science has shown can be helpful (*see chapter 5 for more details*). There is not a shred of scientific evidence for any quick-fix approach that guarantees you more than this. If there were, we promise we would tell you.

Most quick-fix solutions are unhelpful for most people

We have listed plenty of reasons why quick-fix 'diets' are not the way forward. However, on the whole, the diet industry continues to sell solutions that have all of the problems above – and they are making millions doing it.

We hope to show you a good alternative to all of these problems. Before this, though, there is one final point.

The 'Perfect Diet'

Imagine that we have invented the Perfect Diet. It is flexible, does not ban any foods, is healthy, allows for the occasional treat and will result in steady weight loss. We have made this diet scientifically perfect for you. We know that if you stay with it, you will lose weight.

Imagine that we give you this diet plan, but there are some things that we cannot give you. Imagine that *nothing else in your life changes*. That means:

* You are still the same person.
* You still have the same routine.
* You still have the same family and friends.
* You still have the same emotions and attitudes.

How well would you do?

Here are some things that might happen:

* Old habits of snacking or binging might start again, sometimes with you hardly noticing them.
* Other people could get in the way – either by actively trying to stop you losing weight or by just refusing to be helpful with the Perfect Diet.

- Other parts of your life might get in the way – for example, having to have crisps in for the kids or not really having an area in which you feel safe to go out walking.
- You might not really have good personal reasons to manage your weight but be trying the Perfect Diet because you felt you 'ought' to or because the doctor said so.
- You might not believe that the Perfect Diet – or any new programme – will work.
- You might not believe, deep down, that you can stick to any programme and make it work.
- You might have worries that the programme will fail and you will put on even more weight.
- You might quite enjoy the indulgence and pleasure of breaking the diet.
- You might feel you shouldn't have to do this, that it isn't fair.
- You might break the diet just a little then say, 'I've blown it now', and lose track for days.

Most of us would have problems with some of these, even if we were using the Perfect Diet. Why is this?

The difficulty is that eating and activity happen in our lives – and our lives are often very complicated. It's all very well having the perfect plan, but how can it succeed if our lives are going to get in the way?

All of the changes we have to make to lose weight have to be put into practice in the context of our own unique lives and our own unique set of beliefs and emotions. This might not sound easy, and in most instances it's hard work, but people can do it. It's worth finding out more about these successes.

Weight-loss 'experts'

American scientists have been studying a group of over 10,000 experts in weight loss. This group is called the National Weight Control Registry (NWCR). Here's why they are considered experts:

- All of the people in this group have lost at least 5 stone (30kg) in weight and have kept it off for at least one year, and usually much longer than this.
- They have done this in different ways, and before succeeding most of the group had attempted to lose weight many times in the past. They had lost (and presumably regained) large amounts of weight before they managed to keep it off.
- As well as losing weight, most NWCR members report mood and self-confidence have improved and they have increased levels of energy and mobility.

Clearly, the NWCR group managed to do what thousands of people across the world would love to do and it's helpful to see what can be learned from this group. This was the purpose of setting up the NWCR, so researchers could work out what people who lose weight and keep it off are doing. So, what do we know?

First of all, most of these people had good reasons to lose weight. Over three-quarters of the sample said that some event made them decide to lose weight. This was usually something medical (like back pain or fatigue), or some important emotional event (for example, a relationship breaking down due to weight).

Then the NWCR group changed *both* their eating *and* their activity habits. The most common changes were:

- Eating regularly – on average five times per day
- Eating breakfast
- Changing certain types or classes of foods
- Changing portion sizes
- Focusing on reducing fat

These experts also got very serious about activity. However, the types of activity were just as simple as the changes made to their eating. Most chose one or two activities such as walking, swimming, cycling or going to the gym.

What the experts tell us

The studies of the NWCR group do not give us any magical new ideas about methods of weight loss. However, we think there are some very significant lessons to be learned.

First, it is never too late to try to lose weight. Most of the NWCR group were 'dieting veterans' who had lost and regained a good deal of weight in the past.

Second, the NWCR group were generally happier when they had lost weight. Many people worry they will have to permanently 'starve' themselves to keep weight off and they might be smaller but they would be miserable. This doesn't seem to be the case in the NWCR. Higher levels of confidence and happiness were reported after weight loss. Third, and perhaps most importantly, the NWCR group showed that *changing habits* is the key. What they did was simple, but they managed to keep it going year after year.

So what does 'changing habits' mean?

Most of our lives are made up of habits. When we get up in the morning, our habits start. We either get straight out of bed or groan and hit the 'snooze' button. That's a habit. When we get up, some people put on a dressing gown, some don't. That's a habit, too.

Our habits are so routine we usually don't even think about them. But they can be important. Some people are in the habit of having a fried breakfast, some have cereal and some have nothing. These habits may affect people's weight in the long term.

Here are some important facts about habits:

> • When you are used to a habit, it doesn't seem like a big effort.
> • However, changing a habit is difficult and needs some effort and concentration.
> • After a while, though, it begins to seem like less of an effort. That is because a new habit has been formed.

In terms of managing weight, this means there is good and bad news. First, it will be difficult at the beginning. You will be trying to make new habits and break old ones. This is going to be hard, as anyone who has stopped biting their nails or quit smoking can tell you. However, when the new habit is in place, it will become easier.

There is evidence from the NWCR study to back up this idea. Most of the NWCR group found keeping weight off was easier, or similar to losing weight. Changing their habits was the hard part; once this was done, the new habits just kept themselves going and the weight stayed off!

You may be curious to know how you can do it, too. In this book we will show you how to:

- Change your habits of activity and eating over the long term.
- Have a flexible approach to activity and eating that is healthy and balanced.
- Make all of these changes happen in your own unique life.
- Manage all of this yourself, without having to rely on someone else's ideas or support.

We are going to introduce you to some of the latest ideas on how to change behaviour. We know they work. They all come under the heading of 'cognitive behavioural therapy'.

What is cognitive behavioural therapy?

Cognitive behavioural therapy (CBT) is a form of psychological therapy. Now you may be thinking, 'I need help with my eating, not a shrink!' But CBT is really useful for managing weight. It was originally developed for the treatment of depression, but it has been shown to be a highly effective way of changing lots of different behaviours.

The idea behind CBT is that behaviour is always very closely connected to our thoughts and feelings. So if a person wants to change their habits effectively, they will probably have to change their attitudes and respond to some emotions differently. For example:

A thought: This is hopeless. I'll never lose this weight.

There's just no point trying

might be related to. . .

A *feeling*: Feeling miserable, sad, low, which might be related to. . .

A *physical reaction*: Feeling completely out of energy and craving sweets

which might be related to. . .

A form of *behaviour*: Staying in, not going out, 'comfort eating' with sweets

which might be related to. . .

Everything else *all over again*.

If you understand how all of these things happen, you can begin to change the patterns. CBT shows you the best ways to do this.

There are particular parts of CBT that are important:

- It focuses on feelings, thoughts and behaviour in the here and now – not in childhood, for example.

- It is a teaching approach – it does not aim to 'fix' people by telling them what to do, but by teaching them the skills to 'fix' themselves.
- It is an active approach that focuses on trying things out. The trick is to experiment and see what works.

All of this will become clearer as we go through the book.

How to use this book

What this book is about

This book is about managing weight over the long term to improve health and have the best possible quality of life. It is not primarily about losing weight to look good. We think it's important not to support the idea that everybody should be a 'perfect' size or shape. Many people spend lots of time worrying about their weight, size and shape when they are perfectly healthy. Of course, there's *absolutely nothing wrong* with wanting to look good and the techniques in this book will work just fine to achieve this. But the main aim for changing is to improve health and quality of life.

This book is about changing eating habits *and activity*. They go together. For someone who is serious about managing weight in the long term, neither is optional.

INTRODUCTION

What this book is not about

This book is not about managing eating disorders. Eating disorders (bulimia, anorexia, binge-eating disorder) are serious problems that damage people's lives. There are good books, support services and health services for people with these problems, including some of the other books in this series, for example *Overcoming Bulimia Nervosa and Binge-Eating* by Peter Cooper, *Overcoming Binge Eating* by Christopher Fairburn or *Overcoming Anorexia Nervosa* by Patricia Graham and Christopher Freeman.

- If you are binging and then vomiting or using laxatives regularly – for example, every week – please go to your doctor. Many overweight people have vomited once or twice in their lives in order to lose weight, but this doesn't mean that they have bulimia. It is time to be concerned if you are still doing this regularly.
- If your BMI is below 20 (see page 361) then this book is not for you. Losing even more weight will hurt you. It will not make you happier. There are people who have the skills and knowledge to help you with this difficulty. Please use the services that are available to you and speak to your doctor.

How this book is organised

We have written this book to a very clear plan, but we realise that people will read it in different ways. Some people might prefer to read the sections that seem most useful and skip the rest. Others will start at page 1 and read slowly and thoroughly to the end. There is no right or wrong way to do it. However, we wrote the book in a particular way, and it is useful for you to know why.

The book is written in two stages:

Part One – chapters 1, 2 and 3 – provides the foundations. It aims to get you motivated, to remove mental blocks and to help you understand your habits. These are hugely useful skills that can be used in all sorts of situations.

Chapter 1 shows you how to work out your motivation and includes ideas about what is bad for motivation – for example, guilt.

However, even if a person has motivation, they still might not believe that they are really capable of losing weight. So it is important to work with thoughts and beliefs (chapter 2). Some patterns of thinking can undermine our motivation and confidence.

Finally, before a person can get started with real change, they have to understand their own habits of eating and activity. This is covered in chapter 3.

Part Two – chapters 4 to 9 – is about how to make the changes in your life.

Chapters 4 and 5 explain tried and tested ways to bring

activity into your life and to eat healthily and well for the long term.

However, knowing how to do something is not the same as being able to do it. Chapter 6 covers the 'how to' of changing your routines and habits.

When you make some changes, difficult emotions (for example sadness) or physical feelings (hunger or cravings) may come up. Chapter 7 talks about how to work with these.

Also, other people may not be very supportive when you want to make changes. Chapter 8 covers how to get partners, friends and others on side when you can, and what to do when you are not getting the support you need.

Finally, Chapter 9 sums everything up and shows you how to plan for the future.

Getting started

You will need to have somewhere to write things down. Many people use a notebook or somewhere on their phone or laptop. You need to be able to express yourself honestly, so make sure whatever method you choose is confidential if you need it to be.

Work out how overweight you are

It's also a good idea to learn how professionals calculate health risks linked to being overweight. They use a particular measure known as body mass index, or BMI. BMI is just a measure of weight that takes account of height.

You can calculate your own BMI using the table in Appendix I (page 361) or there are plenty of online BMI calculators for you to try.

So, what does this number mean? Here are the classifications that professionals use:

19.9 or less	Underweight	Should not be losing weight
20–24.9	Healthy weight	Should keep weight stable
25–29.9	Overweight	Health at risk from weight
30–39.9	Obese	Health at high risk from weight
40+	Morbidly obese	Health at very high risk

BMI gives you an idea about whether you may be at greater risk of various health conditions (such as diabetes, high blood pressure or heart disease), although there are many other factors apart from body size that determine health (e.g. smoking, sleep, stress). If your BMI is high, it isn't necessary to lower it to an 'ideal' or 'optimal' level, but instead to focus on making changes to eating and activity habits because these influence health and support managing weight.

We hope this book helps you to enjoy food more, not less, by taking the stress, uncertainty and guilt out of eating. Likewise, that activity is no longer seen as a chore, or too intimidating to even consider. Taking the approach described in this book will help you make healthier choices around eating, and activity a part of your life. Good luck, we hope you enjoy the journey!

CHAPTER SUMMARY

- Many people have tried to lose weight for years by using quick-fix solutions.
- These usually haven't worked and sometimes have left them feeling as if they had no will-power or were lazy.
- However, high body weight is affecting more and more people in our society.
- Modern life tempts us to eat too much tasty food and keeps us inactive.
- Quick-fix diets are not the way forward for most people: they are rigid, short-term and often rely on a 'fad' theory of weight loss.
- However, people can lose weight and keep it off – and it is never too late to try.
- The solution is changing eating and activity habits in the long term.

PART ONE

THE FOUNDATIONS

1

Motivation to change

You've got to be motivated if you want to lose weight! Dieting takes willpower, you know!

There's a lot of talk about 'willpower' when it comes to changing what we eat and our activity levels. Most of it can end up making people feel bad about themselves. If a person has tried to diet many times but always regained the weight, they often end up thinking that they must have no 'willpower' or be really lazy.

In our view, this isn't helpful. How can you call someone who has tried to change using a dozen different diets 'lazy'? The other problem with talk about 'willpower' is it suggests you either magically have it or you don't, and it doesn't tell us much about *how* to change.

It is true that people often lose their commitment to weight loss; the thought of another attempt can be quite daunting. Sometimes we might make a half-effort – that is, we might have a go at a diet but leave out the bits we don't like. Other times, we might drift on and off a diet – for example, we see a new approach in the media that sounds useful, but when we try it, it's too strict, faddy or boring.

Feeling angry at having to lose weight is also quite common – we might feel angry at ourselves for gaining weight, at health professionals who ask us to lose weight but don't provide ways of doing so, or at the food and diet industry that is making money out of yo-yo dieting. There is also the natural tendency to avoid thinking about difficult things. If something can make us unhappy, it can feel a lot safer to push it to the back of our mind and not think about it.

These are all understandable reactions to the process of losing weight. In fact, they are all normal reactions to any situations that might involve challenge and difficulty.

Willpower is only part of the picture

The good news is we know that 1) willpower is only part of the picture, and 2) willpower isn't a magical power but more like a muscle that we can build up, so it can get stronger and stronger.

We can think of willpower as the fuel that helps keep us going whilst we form new a habit, but to light the fuel we need a spark, and that spark is motivation. It's common to have motivation and willpower for some things and not for others. For example, a teenager might be putting little effort into studying for exams. They might avoid doing work or do so little that it makes no difference. They might find excuses for why they are not studying, or complain when they are forced to. However, the same teenager might have a huge passion for football. They might practise in cold wind and driving rain night after night. They might have an incredible knowledge of players and clubs. Does this mean that they have motivation and willpower or not? The answer is yes when they are working towards something that matters to them personally. Otherwise, no. That difference is the focus of this chapter. Experience tells us that if people are motivated to lose weight for important personal reasons, they tend to do well. If they try because they think they 'should', they don't do well at all.

There are ways to discover, or perhaps rediscover, your important personal reasons to lose weight. Even if you think you are a pretty motivated person, or that you have obvious reasons to lose weight, we suggest you read on.

What is motivation?

Different people use the word motivation to mean different things. When we talk about a motivated person we mean someone who:

- Knows their own personal reasons for doing something
- Is not doing something because they 'should' or 'ought to'
- Really wants to do something and is willing to make the effort
- Is ready for a long-term effort and is willing to experience some unpleasant feelings in the short term to get to their goal

- Knows there is no guarantee of success
- Is willing to work on their own – they might get advice and support, but they know they must make the effort themselves
- Knows what they want, why they want it and why it is important to them
- Is able to appreciate the small successes they achieve on the way to accomplishing a bigger goal

On the other hand, a not very motivated person might be someone who:

- Does not have good reasons to make changes
- Isn't clear what steps they need to take to change
- Has lots of different, competing plans
- Isn't confident they can make changes
- Wishes someone would come and fix the problem for them
- Thinks that the excitement or energy of a new challenge or project ('Yeah! Let's do it!') is the same as motivation
- Expects things to work perfectly every time
- Is doing something because their doctor, friends or partner wants them to do it

> • Will not start something unless they are pretty sure they can succeed

We all recognise a bit of ourselves in the second list, particularly when it comes to doing something difficult. But there is some good news here – that doesn't matter at all! The trick is to build up positive reasons to make changes *and* have a clear plan of what to do broken down into manageable steps.

What is motivation made of?

We can have an idea of what motivation looks like but that doesn't help us to be motivated ourselves. We can watch an Olympic gymnast on TV and recognise their skill but that doesn't mean we can do what they do, or indeed want to. For us to be motivated we need:

1. To have important personal reasons for doing it
2. To believe that it is possible to achieve it

If either of these is missing motivation will be low. For example, imagine that I am someone who would love to be an Olympic gymnast and this would mean a lot to me personally. Unfortunately, even if this were true, I still wouldn't be motivated to start training. This is because I don't have number 2, I am being realistic about my capabilities, and it wouldn't be possible for me to be an Olympic gymnast. Knowing this, I am not motivated to start training.

On the other hand, I am perfectly capable of repainting my bathroom, which has needed doing for months. It's obvious that I would be able to do this, so I do have point number 2 this time. The trouble is, I don't have very many good reasons to do it right now. There are lots of other things that are more important to me. This time, I don't have number 1, the important personal reasons. My bathroom is going to remain unpainted for quite a long time.

So, in order to succeed at something people need both good reasons to do it and the belief they can. In this section we will deal with the reasons. The belief will be covered in chapters 2 and 3. For now, the focus is on finding good personal reasons for managing your weight.

Reasons for losing weight

You may be thinking your reasons for losing weight are pretty obvious. You want to look better, be healthier and be more mobile. Also, it can be really hard to live in a society where people who are overweight are judged. But 'obvious' reasons don't always lead to action. A good example is this man who had an excellent understanding of the health risks of being overweight:

> *My family has a history of diabetes. I know I need to lose weight – I've seen what diabetes can do to people. If you don't control it properly, you can end up going blind or having*

your limbs amputated! I know all of this stuff, but it doesn't seem to make me want to lose weight. It just doesn't make any difference when I've got the food in front of me.

Most of us would think that a health risk as serious as diabetes that can result in amputation or blindness would motivate us to take action. Unfortunately, it doesn't always work like this. Not all reasons give a person real emotional energy, even if they seem important.

One of the problems is that these health risks can seem a long way off in the future, especially compared to making a very immediate choice about what to eat or whether to go out for a walk in the rain. Also, we are remarkably adaptable. So even if someone is finding their life increasingly limited by their weight, for example if their mobility gets worse or they have had another heart attack, these do not necessarily mean that they will make changes. Some people will, some people won't, and a lot of this comes down to how important *and* how achievable losing weight feels.

In order to understand the kind of mental and emotional energy and commitment that's needed, we are going to step away from weight management for a moment. Weight management is a difficult task. But we have all done difficult things in our lives. How did we achieve them?

What reasons can motivate you to do things that are difficult?

Everyone has overcome difficulties at some point in their

lives or made a serious effort at something they didn't have to do. It can be helpful to remember and analyse these times. Whatever gave you the strength then may also give you the strength for weight loss. Try to remember some times when you have done the following:

- Done something difficult that you didn't have to do
- Experienced difficulties and kept going
- Decided to do something that mattered to you, even though you weren't certain you would succeed
- Kept on doing something difficult for a long time
- Been really determined and focused
- Been seen by others to have been really determined or focused

When you have remembered a time like this, try to work out what gave you the energy and kept you going. For many people it was some kind of standard, or ideal, such as 'being a good parent' or 'seeing things through', while for others it was working towards some important goal that they could see 'in the distance'. For example:

- I was determined always to have time for my children, no matter how tired or rushed I was. It's really important for me to be a good parent.
- I've always worked hard at my job and always will. I enjoy doing my work to the best of my ability and delivering a really great service. I love to see customers delighted with what I can give them.
- I kept phoning my friend Paula, as she was going through a rough divorce. It was hard to listen to her at times, but I was determined to be a friend who was there when I was needed.
- I worked hard to get that extra qualification. I was determined to keep developing my own skills and interests. I am the kind of person who keeps learning and I always see things through.
- I'll do any work I have to in order to travel. I scrimped and saved for months to get the money together. You only get one life and there's a huge, beautiful world out there. I'm not going to miss it!

The point of this exercise is to better understand the things that might really matter to you. The name we give these things really doesn't matter – they could be called 'reasons' or 'passions' or 'principles', but we have decided to use 'values'. We may think we know what our values are, but looking back at what has really motivated us in the past can sometimes give us clues about what is important to us, and remind us that we are actually capable of achieving difficult things when they are important to us.

Of course, people change and our lives change, and so does what is important to us.

Helpful ways to think about values

Thinking about what's important to you is a huge topic, so it can be helpful to think about particular areas of your life one at a time. Below are some areas to think about. It's useful to write down what matters to you under each heading. Also, work out *how much* each reason you think of matters to you. Is it something you would barely get out of bed for? Or would you move heaven and earth to achieve it?

This isn't a complete list, of course. If there are other things that matter to you which are not on this list, then please just add them. Conversely, some of these categories may not apply to you at all, so you can ignore them.

- Relationships – your partnerships, in the present or future
- Family – your children, siblings, parents
- Social life – what kind of friend you want to be, how you want your friendships to develop
- Work – your career or vocation, your ambitions

- Education and training – how do you want to develop your mind and skills?
- Recreation – how do you want to spend your leisure time? What's your idea of fun and relaxation?
- Spirituality – however you relate to the meaning of your life, the bigger picture
- Citizenship – your role in society, perhaps 'giving something back'
- Health and wellbeing – how do you want to maintain your health, for example eating, sleep, physical activity, smoking?

When you're doing this, try to be honest. Don't just write what sounds good if that doesn't really feature in your most important priorities. No one else need ever read this list.

Here are some ways to generate more ideas:

- Think of people whose lives or characters you admire.
- Remember the things you used to dream about as a child.
- Imagine yourself as you would like to be. What does this person want out of life? What do they value?

- Imagine you are at your own funeral, hearing people talk about your life. What would you like to hear them saying?
- Find someone who's known you a long time and ask them what they think of as your real passions and values.

Once you have some ideas, write them down. Put everything down, even if it doesn't seem as though it's very helpful for weight loss.

Put your reasons in positive terms

The actual words you use when writing down your values are important. Values are most useful when they are put in positive terms. For example, these are two different ways of seeing the same situation:

I worked two jobs at the same time because we had so little money. It was really hand to mouth – I just had to keep going to pay the bills. I don't know where I found the strength.

I worked two jobs at the same time because we had so little money. I was determined to do what I had to do to keep family life normal. I made sure the kids didn't want for anything and I didn't want to have to disrupt their lives by having to move to a smaller place. I found the strength because I was doing it for them.

Both have the same outcome but the second one phrases things in a more positive light and connects to values. It focuses on what was really important in that situation. In the first example, it may seem that paying bills was the important thing. But that only mattered because unpaid bills would have disrupted family life. Family life was what was really important, so when the person in this example comes to write their reasons down, they should focus on that, as this is an important value to them. Understanding that this is the key motivator and keeping this in mind is going to be helpful when challenges with weight management arise. This leads us on to the next question.

How does managing your weight connect to the things that you value?

The answer to this question may be clear already. Alternatively, there may seem to be no connections at all between what's important to you and weight loss. The next exercise is an imaginative and practical way of joining up what you value with why you want to manage your weight.

The 'Five Years' exercise

It's hard for most of us to get the motivation *now* for things that will benefit us *in the future*. So the 'Five Years' exercise uses your imagination to picture what your life in the future could be and how your weight might affect that.

To do this exercise it is helpful to put aside some time when you won't feel rushed or be interrupted. We would suggest you try to do most of it all at once, but you can always come back to it and add more ideas as you think of them. We would also suggest that you write down your answers to these questions so you have a record of your thoughts. These are quite big questions so it can help to have a record you can return to and reflect upon.

Imagine yourself in five years' time

This may sound a little hard, but you can do it. Imagine two different futures and do them one at a time. First of all, work out:

- How old will you be in five years' time?
- How old will the people who are close to you be?

1. WEIGHT-GAIN FUTURE

In this future, you have lost no weight at all and have even gained some (most adults gain weight over a five-year period). Your health is the same as it is now, or perhaps slightly worse. You may have slightly less energy, more aches and pains, and be slightly less mobile.

Now ask yourself the following questions:

- Where are you likely to be living?
- What will you be doing with your time? What will you be able, or not able, to do?

- What will have happened by then? Pay attention to any big events that you know now will be coming up in the next five years. What will these events have been like?
- Imagine a typical day – getting out of bed and so on. Imagine all of your sensations, including energy, tiredness and pain.
- How will you be feeling about yourself?
- Imagine how others will be feeling about you. Will they be pleased, or worried about you?

Try to imagine this future and make it as realistic as possible.

2. WEIGHT-LOSS FUTURE

In the second future, you are eating healthily, are regularly active and have lost weight. Your general health is better; you feel fitter and have more energy.

Again, ask yourself the same questions:

- Where will you likely be living?
- What will you be doing with your time? What will you be able, or not able, to do?
- What will have happened by then? Pay attention to any big events that you know now will be coming up in the next five years. What will these events have been like?

- Imagine a typical day – getting out of bed and so on. Imagine all of your sensations, including energy, tiredness and pain.
- How will you be feeling about yourself?
- Imagine how others will be feeling about you. Will they be pleased, or worried about you?

INCLUDE THE POSITIVES AND NEGATIVES

When you imagine your two different futures, try to include both positives and negatives. For example, there could be benefits about the weight-gain future. You might have enjoyed not having to think about what you are eating and being able to go with the flow. And in the weight-loss future, perhaps you had to plan more when you didn't feel like it, had less of certain foods you like. Try to really imagine your two futures in as much detail as possible, and to be realistic. Try also to notice any feelings or emotions that come up when you think about these two different futures and make a note of these too.

IN FIVE YEARS' TIME, WILL WEIGHT LOSS REALLY MATTER TO YOU?

What are the important differences between the two futures? And how you feel about them? Think about these differences in terms of the values that you wrote down above and write these differences down framed in a positive way. If you can see that weight loss will affect the things that matter to you, then this will be the fuel for your motivation. If not, things will be trickier but not impossible.

The 'Five Years' exercise was important for **Jackie**:

I'm currently thirty-eight years old, and my son, Craig, is ten. The first thing that comes into my mind when I think about the next five years is my age! I will have had my fortieth birthday and I suppose I will be in my mid-forties. That's a funny thought. When it comes to health, I've always believed, somehow, that people in their forties need to be more careful than people in their thirties. It just sounds older. Craig will be fifteen. I can't imagine him that old, but I suppose by that time he will be wanting to spend a lot less time with me. He'll probably be wanting to see less of the family altogether.

My husband, John, will be five years on into his career. He will hopefully have been promoted. Unfortunately, that will mean he'll probably be working even longer hours so I may see less of him. We will probably still go on holidays together. In fact, that may be the best time I get with them. We will do our usual walking holidays – hills and pub meals are what we enjoy. I do love my food, and we all do as a family. If I got diabetes, that would seriously cramp my style! I would have to be loads more careful about what I ate, and I wouldn't enjoy having to do that under threat of bad health. I'm a nurse, and I've seen lots of diabetes up close. The walking is one area in which my weight bothers me. I'm going to have to be a lot fitter and lighter on my feet than I am now if I'm going

47

to keep up with John and a fifteen-year-old boy. I refuse to be left behind by them.

My plan has always been to get back into nursing as Craig gets older. I was heading for a pretty senior post when I left. It will take me a while to get back to this. I would feel better as a nurse if I was carrying less weight. I probably won't have to do too much physical stuff any more, but I would feel better about leading a team of nurses if I were fitter and lighter. It's just the way I feel about my role.

So, I will sum up like this. I am going to have more time to develop myself in the next five years. I can make a decision about which way my weight goes. My love of food actually makes me want to lose weight – I couldn't bear to find out I was diabetic. I'd hate to watch what I eat because of that. I would also like to be fitter as I refuse to be left behind physically by the boys! Finally, I'd feel happier as a senior nurse if I was carrying less weight. So losing weight is important in a lot of ways – for family life, self-development, career and holidays. I don't think that knowing this will make it easy, but at least my priorities are clear.

Jackie found lots of important reasons for losing weight, but other people come up with very different answers:

My weight doesn't stop me from doing my evening courses or going to my book group. On the other hand,

I would be annoyed if I hadn't got control of my weight in the next five years. As far as I'm concerned, I am a determined and organised person, and I should be able to make things like that happen.

I'm not sure my weight makes any difference to the things I really want. It doesn't stop me from travelling — and most of the places I go, people are a lot more relaxed about weight than here! And I'm pretty active, and not too overweight, so my health isn't really a problem.

I'm a bit stuck — I can't work out what weight has to do with the important things in my life.

Don't worry if it doesn't all seem to be going to plan. People often get stuck at this point or find that they have some of the following problems:

- I'm in two minds about this — either having lots of good reasons but still not wanting to lose weight, or not having any good reasons but still wanting to lose weight.
- Some of the things that matter to me would make me less likely to lose weight!
- I just can't see any personally important reasons to lose weight.

We will think through all of these problems in the following sections.

What to do with things that reduce your motivation

Being in two minds – or even having good reasons not to lose weight

It's very common for people to have some good personal reasons to lose weight and some good personal reasons not to. For example, a person might have these two reasons:

1. To stay healthy so they can enjoy life and time with their family
2. To live for the moment and not worry about tomorrow

This person might be faced with a bit of a contradiction. 'Staying healthy' would involve managing their eating and physical activity, and 'living for the moment' would suggest the opposite!

Here is another example. A person might have these two reasons:

1. To lose weight so I feel better about the way I look and so I can be more active
2. To not judge people by how big they are or their weight

It's obviously wrong to judge a person by their weight. So this person might ask, 'Why am I judging *myself* by my own weight? Why do I need to lose weight at all?' They might find that the second reason gives them *less* motivation to lose weight.

These are important issues. If mixed feelings are there, it is important to be open about them. However, we can often think about mixed feelings or 'demotivating' reasons in a way that sorts them out – at least a little. It's helpful to do two things: check that your reasons are 'demotivating' and work against weight loss, and then decide on your 'trade-offs'.

Check that the reasons really do work against weight loss

Take, for example, 'living for the moment', and 'not judging people by their weight'. It seems that both of these ideas work against weight loss. But do they really?

This is an important question, because a lot of the time these 'difficult' reasons are not what they seem.

You can ask two useful questions about reasons like these:

1. Do they actually oppose weight loss when you think about it?
2. Are you sure they really have anything to do with weight loss at all?

For example, if a person wants to 'live for the moment', does that really mean they cannot achieve weight loss? Losing weight needs a long-term commitment. It means that a person must think about what they eat and how active they are *today* if they are going to control what they will weigh *in the future*. So if a person wants to live *absolutely* for the moment, and eat what they like, and do as little activity as they feel like at the moment – then yes, this reason will not help with weight loss.

On the other hand, is a person really able to 'live for the moment' if they have back pain? Is it easy to be spontaneous when you have to remember to take your medication for blood pressure or diabetes? How can you 'live for the moment' if you can't really keep up with your children or friends because you are not fit enough? So, thinking it through, this reason actually can encourage weight loss.

How about 'not judging people by their weight'? Most people would hopefully agree that a person's weight has nothing to do with whether they are kind, honest, intelligent or a valuable person, but however lovely a person is, the very real health risks of being seriously overweight will still exist. So this is an example of how a reason that seems to work against weight loss actually has nothing at all to do with weight.

Decide on your trade-offs, and be honest about what you will lose

Of course, even when you think things through, there might still be 'trade-offs'. This is not something to worry about. Everyone knows that almost every serious decision in life has both pluses and minuses. Thinking these through clearly can help you make an informed decision about them.

For example, the person who wants to 'live for the moment' is going to have to make a choice between eating what they like when they like and doing as little physical activity as they like and being healthy enough to be free and spontaneous in the future.

Looking at trade-offs means being really clear about the costs and benefits of losing weight. There are nearly always costs. People almost always have to make changes to long-term patterns of eating. They also might have to increase their amount of physical activity, even if this isn't their favourite thing. Think hard now about everything that would be difficult about weight loss. Will you go through all that to get the rewards?

Please note! If the hard things seem absolutely terrible, then it is probably worth doing this exercise again after you have read the next two chapters.

Your reasons for change are something you can come back to when times get tough, and also add to when you are doing well and reaping the rewards. Don't worry if it's not all worked out right now.

There is one last thing to do with your reasons. Some reasons are guaranteed to leave you in two minds or not make you feel good. It's best to get rid of them altogether.

Throw out the guilt

Changing something because of guilt, because we feel we ought to or should do something, is unlikely to work in the long term. In fact it might have the opposite effect.

Guilt might get you started but it won't keep you going in the long term. Because guilt is a negative emotion we might end up trying to avoid thinking about what is making us feel guilty. So if weight loss is about guilt, we will start avoiding thinking about weight loss. The other thing about guilt is it can often lead to the very thing we are trying to avoid, like overeating. We will talk more about this in chapter 7.

It might be that you can change your guilty reasons so they are positive. For example, if you change 'I shouldn't be so careless about my health' to 'I choose to look after my health because it matters to me and my family', does it sound any more motivating?

So where are you now?

You have now had some time and space to consider how managing your weight connects to what is important to you now and in the future. You can use the following questions to help pull all this together:

1. Are your reasons really personal and connected to the values that matter in your life?
2. Have you written them down?

3. Have you written them down in positive terms?
4. Is weight loss something that is important to your life?
5. Have you noticed any 'shoulds' or 'ought tos' or guilt and questioned the value of these?
6. Have you considered the trade-offs involved?

At this point you are likely to have either mostly found some important and convincing reasons to lose weight or you haven't. Which one applies to you?

1. You have found some important personal reasons to motivate you

If you have good reasons to lose weight then you are more likely to get off to a good start and keep going when things get tricky.

There is one problem: reasons are easy to forget. And when we forget them, we tend to lose energy and determination. So it's important to try to find a way to remember, starting with writing them down, if you haven't already.

Then you need to put them somewhere where you can look at them regularly. If you prefer a big public statement, you could stick them on your fridge door. If your reasons are more of a private thing, you could keep them in your wallet or purse. Or you could set a reminder on your computer or phone so they pop up regularly. How do you usually remember things? Whatever way you decide, the important thing is you have *your* reasons, in *your* words, in a place where you can see them regularly. Reconnecting to your values will provide the emotional 'spark' for your journey.

2. You have not found enough good reasons, or your reasons don't really seem motivating

If you have completed the exercises above and have found that losing weight does not connect to what you value in your life now or looking forward to the future then this might not be the best time for you to try to manage your weight. However, you might find it helpful to make a note to redo the exercises in six months' or a year's time in case things have changed. It is also important to remember that even if you decide you don't have the reasons or motivation to lose weight at the moment you might still consider some small changes that could benefit your health, for example adjusting the types of food you are eating or increasing the amount of activity you're doing. The following chapters can help you to make those changes so it might be worth reading on.

CHAPTER SUMMARY

- We can think of willpower as the fuel that helps keep us going whilst we form new a habit, but to light the fuel we need a spark.

- The spark is motivation; it helps us get started and keeps us going through the challenging times.

- Motivation consists of two things: having important personal reasons to do something and believing we can do it.

- Connecting what we value in our lives to important personal reasons for managing our weight is key for motivation.

- It is normal to be 'in two minds' about weight loss and to have doubts. Understanding these can help us be clearer about why we want to change and to overcome difficulties.

- Motivation through guilt does not work in the long term. If possible, try to make your reasons positive and throw out the 'shoulds'.

- If now does not feel like the time to try to manage your weight, are there any small changes that you could make that would benefit your health or wellbeing?

- Remembering and reconnecting to our values on a regular basis can help reignite our spark when the going gets tough.

2

Thoughts and beliefs

You've got to think positively if you want to lose weight. Stop being so negative!

Many people agree that the way a person thinks about managing weight will affect how successful they are. Although there is unlikely to be one 'perfect' attitude, we are convinced some patterns of thinking are unhelpful and may impact negatively on results.

We can all look around us and see people whose attitudes seem to make their attempts to change less likely to work. Some people never try new challenges because they are sure that they won't succeed. Others are so convinced they are unattractive that they avoid romance and push people away when they seem interested. You can probably think of many examples like this.

Patterns of thinking can often make difficult situations worse. Although it's easy to say, 'Think positively', it's often difficult to know how to go about it. Also, you need to recognise there is something unhelpful about your thinking in the first place. One of the great benefits of CBT is it shows you, in practical ways, how to check if your thinking patterns are helping or hindering and how to make changes if helpful.

However, before we start, let's be clear about which kinds of thinking are important for weight management. After all, the word 'thinking' could be applied to doing a difficult crossword, or daydreaming in the shower, or taking a penalty kick. These are all very different mental processes!

'Automatic' thinking patterns

To get an idea of which types of thinking are important for weight loss, take a look at **Pete's** thinking patterns. Pete is trying to eat healthily but is very busy at work and due to give an important presentation later on this morning.

The alarm goes off. . .

Oh, God, I feel like I've just gone to sleep. I haven't had enough sleep to cope with this presentation. I need to jump in the shower before I drop off again. I wish this presentation was another day. Actually, I wish Sue could have done it, she's better at this kind of thing. I wish I had her confidence, it would make the presentation so much easier. I should stick to desk work and let other people do the public speaking.

Breakfast. . . Cereal and fruit juice. Oh, how depressing. On a morning like this, I could really do with a fry-up! Just when I need some energy for the day I'm only allowed to have cereal. . .

Looking at the children's lunchboxes. . .

This really isn't helping me. Having crisps in the house for the kids means I end up eating them just because they're there. If it's in the house, I will always eat it. . .

Dressed and ready to leave the house. . .

Well, at least I look OK for the presentation. Well sort of . . . look at that belly. It would all be different if I could get some exercise. I could be really fit, and I'd have loads more energy. I wish I could be fitter. . .

All of the time between waking up and going to work, Pete was thinking. He was doing things the whole time and he was having different feelings (feeling nervous and stressed, for example), but he was constantly thinking: about the future (mainly worrying); about himself (not being very confident and having a big stomach); and about what is fair and what is allowed (he wasn't 'allowed' a fried breakfast). There were plans, too (to exercise), and he was trying to work out the causes of his problems (having crisps around the house).

Pete had not decided to sit down and think about his life that morning. In fact, he was hardly aware that he was having these thoughts – they were just running through his mind, like having a radio on in the background. This is the way that our minds work much of the time. So, lots of important thinking happens automatically and we often hardly notice that we are doing it.

Unfortunately, we are usually not able to notice that our thoughts are just thoughts – we assume they are true. This can be a serious problem in managing weight – and for many other parts of life. It's only when something happens to jolt us out of our assumptions that we are able to see that it's just our minds making judgements or having opinions.

All of our thinking could be put somewhere in the boxes below:

Thoughts are true!		Thoughts are just thoughts
Thoughts are completely automatic.	⇔	Person has the thought, but realises that it's just another thing going through their heads.
Person does not realise it's just a thought. It just seems like the truth.	⇔	They realise that there are probably other ways of thinking about the situation.
Person is not able to see any alternatives.	⇔	They can see the beginning of an emotional reaction to the thought, but aren't caught up in this.
The thought can provoke strong emotions or reactions.		

Most of us spend our lives on the left-hand end of this. This is not necessarily a problem. Lots of thinking is automatic, and that's the way that it's meant to be. It wouldn't help if we tried to analyse our thoughts every moment of the day. However, we are particularly likely to be at the left-hand end of the line if we are stressed or sad. At these times it seems that thoughts – particularly negative thoughts – are very definitely true. And this can get us into trouble.

The rest of this chapter focuses on how to move thinking to the right-hand end of the line. At the right-hand end there is more freedom, and there are more choices in our feelings and habits.

How automatic thinking can get us into trouble

Automatic thinking can be useful, but it can also make difficult situations worse and cause all sorts of unpleasant emotions. It may lead us to behave in ways we regret later on or take us away from what we hope to achieve. We can work through some of Pete's thoughts to see how they affected his mood:

- Is Pete really bad at presentations? Would he have been picked for such an important job if he was no good at it?
- Does he really need to avoid the presentation? Might it be an opportunity to practise his skills?
- Does he really need a fry-up? Or does he really need to feel less nervous?
- Is it true that he's not allowed a fry-up? Who is stopping him from having one?
- Is having crisps in the house for the kids part of Pete's problem? It might be. But could he do something about this rather than just feeling defeated about it?

> • Similarly, Pete might well be right about exercise – he could be fitter and have more energy. Could he make time to think about this and make a plan rather than just imagining everything would be perfect if he went to the gym?

Pete's thinking wasn't helping him cope with his nerves or manage his weight. It is important to recognise it was his automatic, moment-by-moment thinking that was the problem. His conscious mind was very clear – he was trying to keep to his healthy plan. He also knew he had managed difficult presentations at work before. Unfortunately, when stressed, these were not the only thoughts going through his head. The automatic thoughts were there, too.

Strong emotions and serious difficulties change automatic thinking

Automatic thoughts are often problematic when strong emotions or 'stuck' habits are present. Here are three ways in which automatic thinking goes wrong.

1. THOUGHTS ARE BIASED OR UNTRUE

Automatic thinking often puts a negative 'spin' on events, e.g. Pete's prediction his presentation would go badly. It's the type of thinking that convinces people that managing weight is hopeless or that they don't have the willpower to succeed.

Common styles of automatic thinking about managing weight include:

- All or nothing – for example, a person might think, 'I'm doing fantastically – I've stuck to my plan,' before thinking, 'I've screwed it up completely. I may as well give up.'
- Catastrophic – believing things will always go wrong. 'This new plan will be like the rest – lots of effort and deprivation and then the weight will go back on.'
- Focusing on the negatives and ignoring the positives – for example, concentrating on the one 'slip' in the week and ignoring the gym sessions they had attended.
- Self-blaming – for example, 'I'm so stupid. I've got no willpower. Why can't I manage to lose weight?' In this style, the person takes something that is genuinely difficult, perhaps even unavoidable, and blames themselves, often believing it's due to a flaw in their own character.

All of these are classic styles of biased or untrue automatic thoughts. There are many more. You may recognise some in yourself already.

2. THEY ARE UNHELPFUL

Of course, automatic thinking is not always biased, it can be true and still be very unhelpful. Take, for example, the thought, 'I've never yet managed to lose weight and keep it off.' This might be quite true. But does it really help? What would it do for someone's mood or motivation?

3. THEY HAVE A LIMITED PERSPECTIVE

We know people tend to think their automatic thoughts are true. There's also a tendency to believe they are the *only* truth. This is often not the case.

Taking 'I've never yet managed to lose the weight and keep it off' as an example, consider some alternative views:

> *I've not had much luck losing weight before, but each time I've learned a bit more about what doesn't work. I've never tried to lose weight with this method before.*
>
> *This is a completely new thing for me.*
>
> *It doesn't necessarily matter if I lose much weight. This time I'm going to focus on my fitness, because it's so important for my health.*
>
> *I know research says it can take a few attempts before finding an approach that suits me. It took me three times to pass my driving test!*

There are many alternative ways to view the same situation, and different parts of the situation to focus on.

It's not just 'negative thinking' that is a problem

Although thinking positively sounds like a good idea, it may not help in really difficult situations. First, it ignores that positive thoughts can be unhelpful, and crucially doesn't tell us *how* to change our thinking.

Take the thought: 'If I just follow this fantastic new diet I will easily lose lots of weight and keep it off!' Is this thought 'negative'? No, it's very positive but it's probably untrue and unhelpful because it encourages wishful thinking.

As we go through the chapter, we will show you how to spot unhelpful thinking – and more importantly, how to see it for what it is and change it.

Becoming more aware of automatic thinking

Our automatic thoughts can help to keep us stuck in old habits and emotions, but as we become more aware of the impact of automatic thinking on our lives, our options increase and change will be easier.

The skills presented in the following sections of the book will allow you to be more aware of your thinking habits. You will start to realise what is bothering you and holding you back. To get started, it is useful to have a look at some common negative thoughts about weight. Then we can learn how to spot them.

What automatic thoughts look like

Teaching a person to see their own thinking is a bit like

66

teaching a new gardener how to identify a rare type of plant. The gardener needs lots of examples of what the plant looks like and they also need to know where it usually lives. This is the approach we will follow here.

Have a look at the following examples. These are common thoughts in people who are trying to manage weight. Some of them may be familiar to you, some not. You will certainly have many more examples. It is important to note that these automatic thoughts are usually some kind of *statement about how things are or how they should be.*

Some examples of automatic thoughts about weight loss

Remember, these are not necessarily untrue, but they are often biased, unhelpful, or only take a limited view of the situation.

Thoughts about what caused the weight problem

I don't understand why I've gained weight. I don't eat all day.

I don't understand why my weight has increased. I don't eat more than my friend, and she's slim.

I may have a problem with my metabolism/my glands/ the way my body stores fat.

Thoughts on what to do about the problem and what this 'solution' will be like

Losing weight will be awful – I'll be hungry/miserable/deprived all of the time.

My life is busy and difficult enough already. I can't cope with losing weight at the same time.

Losing weight will be horrible. I'll have to go running and do aerobics.

I don't want to spend my life counting calories or going to the gym every day.

I won't be able to go out and eat with my friends.

My weight is so high, I've got such a long way to go. It's too much. I just can't face it. I can't imagine getting there.

I've got such a lot of weight to lose. I must be really strict and stop eating all snacks.

Even if I lose loads of weight I will still be big.

Thoughts about what you 'can' and 'can't' do

I can't bear feeling hungry and I hate exercise.

I can't do this. I've tried every diet in the book and they've all failed.

I can't do this. I never stick to any new regime. I'm just fundamentally weak-willed.

I can't do this. I have a problem with food. Something is seriously wrong and needs fixing.

I can't exercise until I feel better about my body.

I can't change until my self-esteem improves.

I can eat this now, I'll exercise more tomorrow.

I've worked really hard all day. I can give myself this treat.

It's raining outside, I can go for a longer walk tomorrow.

Thoughts about what you should and shouldn't do, and what is fair and what isn't

I shouldn't have to do this — it's not fair.

I should be able to eat what I like — other people can eat what they like and stay slim.

I shouldn't have to do this — it's not fair that just eating what I like makes me gain weight.

I shouldn't have to change — other people should accept me just as I am.

I should be able to just do this. I'm just such a failure.

Thoughts that happen 'on the spot' whilst trying to manage weight

I've just blown my plan. I may as well give up now.

I hate this. I want to eat right now, and I'm not allowed to.

I hate this. I don't want to spend my whole life controlling myself.

If I eat just a little of what I want, I will lose control and ruin everything.

I've just finished a really difficult piece of work, I deserve this treat.

I've just had a miserable time, I need something to pick myself up.

I've just done really well! That was fantastic! I deserve this.

I'll worry about weight later. I'm not going to think about it now.

I'm not going to let a stupid diet tell me what to do, I'm going to eat this.

I don't care. I'm going to eat this.

Food is one of the great joys in life. Why would I want to deny myself?

Thoughts about yourself

I'm pathetic. I can't believe I let it get this bad. I deserve to be this weight.

My body is disgusting. I'm repulsive.

I have stuck to my programme, so I am a good person.

I have not stuck to my programme, so I am a bad person.

I'm weak-willed/lazy/stupid.

Now you have a flavour of some of the biased, limited and unhelpful thoughts that get in the way of weight loss, we will get on to spotting some of your own thinking.

Where automatic thoughts tend to live

Being able to spot or 'catch' an automatic thought is a hugely useful skill. However, it is not easy or straightforward. Like the gardener trying to spot the rare plant, it takes practice – and a little bit of good advice. We have already shown you what some automatic thoughts look like and now we will show you where they live!

Unhelpful automatic thoughts live in all sorts of places, but are nearly always found:

- Near strong feelings like sadness, fear, shame and anger
- Near strong physical sensations like hunger, feeling full, feeling tired or feeling deprived
- Near changes in feeling – for example, going from feeling calm to being a little tense or from happy to a little bit sad
- Near issues and habits that are 'stuck' and difficult to change

Follow your feelings

The rule here is *follow your feelings*. When you feel strong emotions or strong physical feelings, that is where you will find the most important automatic thoughts. Here are some example situations:

Deciding that you should probably start a weight-management programme

Deciding that you look big or unfit

Looking at 'weight' material – diet books, magazines, etc.

Seeing pictures of slim people or people who seem to be able to eat lots and maintain their weight

Being tempted to eat something that isn't part of your plan

Just after overeating

Starting a weight-management programme

Trying to exercise and finding it difficult

Looking at a meal that seems to be a 'small' amount of 'healthy' food

Thinking about past attempts to manage weight

Think about the past twenty-four hours. You have probably had some kind of feelings about your weight during this time – if you're really stuck, think how some of the material in this book has made you feel! You can go back beyond the last twenty-four hours if you like but try to think of a recent situation. Once you've decided on a recent situation of feeling, we can work out the linked automatic thoughts and how to deal with them.

Pinpointing the most important automatic thoughts

The next step is to put your finger on the most upsetting part of the situation and put it into words. Use your notebook here – you will need to write this all down, as it won't all fit in your head!

To get to the main automatic thoughts, you can ask these questions about your upsetting situation:

> What was going through my mind just before I started to feel this way?
>
> What does this say about me? What does it say I can/can't do?
>
> What does this mean about me? My life? My future?
>
> What am I afraid might happen? What is the worst thing that could happen if this is true?

What does this mean about what other people might think/feel about me?

What does this mean I should/shouldn't do?

What images or memories do I have in this situation?

Write down some answers to these questions. You may find there is just one main answer or there are lots. There can be dozens of confusing thoughts in any situation. We need to be able to cut through all of the confusion and focus on the most important issue. There are two steps to 'pinpointing' the thought:

1. Explain what the worse part of the problem, situation or emotion is.
2. Summarise it briefly.

This process will allow you get straight to the heart of the matter.

STEP 1: EXPLAINING THE THOUGHT

Remember the rule: 'Follow the feeling.' It is most useful to focus on the thought that has the most emotion attached to it or the one that seems most personally important and meaningful. However, it can be hard to write this down in a way that helps. Some of the time we can look at a situation and realise that our thoughts were things like:

Oh no! Not again!
I can't bear this! That idiot!

Catching these thoughts is great, but we need to go a step deeper than this and work out exactly what the problem is. For example, if the thought is 'Oh no!' then what exactly is wrong? If the thought is 'I can't bear it!' then what exactly is it that the person can't bear? If it's 'That idiot!' what exactly did the idiot do and why does it matter? It's important to explain the issues.

For example, when the unclear thought 'I can't bear it!' was pinpointed, the thought was actually: 'I can't bear the thought of struggling with another diet and failing again!'

This was an example of a thought that was really too short or unclear. Of course, the problem can also run in the opposite direction. A person can try to write down a thought and end up writing pages and pages, so. . .

STEP 2: SUMMARISE THE MAIN ISSUE

Remember, the point of this exercise is to explain and summarise the most important or upsetting aspect of a situation or feeling. If you try to write down your thought but you find that you are writing a lot, then you can probably pinpoint even further. For example:

It's really a problem. Nothing has ever helped me lose weight. I have tried everything over a period of years and I'm completely stuck. None of the diets seem to work. I've no idea if I am ever going to shift this problem.

This can probably briefly be summarised as:

Nothing has ever worked before and nothing ever will work.

Here is another example:

Diets just don't suit me. Or I'm not suited to diets. Each time I've tried it has simply been torment. I've ended up thinking about food every second of the day. I just don't know how I'm going to get around this. I don't want my entire life to be wrapped up in food and calories.

This can be summarised as:

Weight loss will be unpleasant and spoil my everyday life.

Remember, the skill here is to quickly and effectively pinpoint the heart of the problem – or what you think is the heart of the problem. This will be your main automatic thought.

How did it feel?

If you are still having difficulties working out the automatic thoughts in your upsetting situation, try holding the situation in mind and remembering exactly what it felt like. Then ask yourself how you would have completed these sentences at that time:

I am ....

I am not ....

I can ....

I can't ....

The future is ....

I should ....

I should not ....

Other people are ....

My problems with weight are caused by ....

What I need to do is ....

If I try to lose weight, the process will be ....

Remember, as you complete these statements, we are not looking for your 'sensible', clever answers. The most important thing is to recognise how your mind works automatically in difficult and 'stuck' situations. We need to work with your automatic mind, not your sensible mind, if change is going to happen.

What you can do about unhelpful thinking patterns

Now that you have found one or more important automatic thoughts, you need to deal with them. There are two steps:

1. Question the thought.
2. Expand your thinking.

It is not always true that a thought – even a negative one attached to a strong emotion – is biased or untrue. The way to find out whether a thought is true is to question it.

The second step is to expand your thinking. As we noted earlier, even if thoughts are true, they usually only put across one view of a situation. Expanding your thinking is about getting more views and therefore more options for change.

Step 1: How to question the thought

If you have found a thought that is attached to a strong negative emotion or a 'stuck' habit, then this thought needs to explain itself! It needs to be able to convince you that it is being truthful and helpful.

You can imagine that you are a lawyer in a courtroom. The thought is like someone you are cross-examining – someone you are fairly suspicious of. Basically, you want to know 1) if the thought is biased or untrue and 2) if it is helpful or unhelpful.

When you are more practised at this, you will be able to do it quite quickly. To begin with, you will benefit from using the following (and in Appendix I) list of questions that are guaranteed to test any thought in existence.

TOP 10 QUESTIONS FOR THOUGHTS

1. What is the evidence for this thought? What is the evidence against it?
2. What are some other ways of thinking about this situation?

3. How would another person see this situation? What would I say to my best friend or someone I loved if they were in the same situation?

4. What are the advantages and disadvantages of thinking this way?

5. When I am not feeling this way, do I think about this type of situation differently? How?

6. Am I asking questions that have no answers?

7. Five years from now, if I look back at this situation, will I look at it any differently? Will I pay attention to other parts of the situation that I'm ignoring now?

8. Are there any small things that show my thoughts aren't true? Am I ignoring them or not taking them seriously?

9. Am I blaming myself for something over which I do not have complete control? Am I forgetting that other people are responsible for their own behaviour (and I'm not responsible for what they do)?

10. Am I always thinking that things will go badly? Am I exaggerating how bad things would be if they did go wrong?

These questions may not mean much without an example, so here is one from someone you have already met – **Pete**.

Later in the day Pete did his presentation. It went quite well, although he was terribly nervous. He bought himself a doughnut and a packet of crisps to celebrate. Afterwards he became depressed about his weight. He spent some time trying to pinpoint what had made his mood drop after eating the doughnut. He decided the thought was: 'I will never manage to stick to any plan.' Pete was pretty sure that this was true. However, he decided to follow the advice in this book and question the thought anyway. Here are the results of his efforts:

What is the evidence for and against this thought?

Well, I suppose the evidence for this thought is I have never managed it before. Although there have been plenty of difficult things in my life I have finally managed to do. Most people try to stop smoking a few times before they finally manage it. The evidence against it is that I have surprised myself before – done more than I thought I could.

What are some other ways of thinking about this situation?

First, eating a doughnut and a packet of crisps does not mean I am doomed never to lose weight. Second, I could see things as opportunities to learn, rather than just think that I will fail – each time I try to lose weight I learn a little bit more. Third, this way of thinking really gets me down. I am fed up with all the doom and gloom about weight. I'd like to try thinking something else. Fourth, I'm still in good health. I'm a young man – there is plenty of time to keep trying.

How would another person see this situation? What would I say to my best friend or someone I loved if they were in the same situation?

I would encourage a good friend not to give up. I would tell them that managing weight is difficult, but they've done lots of other difficult things in their lives.

What are the advantages and disadvantages of thinking this way?

Advantages? None. Although I suppose if I expect the worst then I won't be so disappointed if it happens. The disadvantages are obvious. I call myself a failure before I have even started. It knocks down my motivation and makes me feel hopeless.

When I am not feeling this way, do I think about this type of situation differently? How?

When I feel less miserable, then I am a bit more optimistic. I have more faith in myself and believe that managing weight is at least possible.

Am I asking questions that have no answers?

A little. This thought can't have an answer because it is about the future. And I have no idea what might happen in the future.

Five years from now, if I look back at this situation, will I look at it any differently? Will I pay attention to other parts of the situation that I'm ignoring now?

Well, I suppose that depends whether I have lost any

weight in five years' time! Actually, maybe not. Whether I have lost weight or not, I will certainly wish I had spent less time telling myself that I was bound to fail. It's a real waste of time, whatever happens.

Are there any small things that show my thoughts aren't true? Am I ignoring them or not taking them seriously?

Maybe. I didn't follow all my plans, but I still had a healthy breakfast and a long walk in the evening. To be honest I'm not sure I even tasted the doughnut and crisps as I ate them so quickly, and once I thought I'd blown it that's when things went downhill with my eating.

Am I blaming myself for something over which I do not have complete control? Am I forgetting that other people are responsible for their own behaviour (and I'm not responsible for what they do)?

Um, this question doesn't seem to apply to this thought.

Am I always thinking that things will go badly? Am I exaggerating how bad things would be if they did go wrong?

Well, I'm certainly not being positive. And what if I did try another weight-loss programme and fail? Does that mean I'm doomed for ever? Not really. It would be a shame, but not a catastrophe.

Pete had felt quite sure that his thought was true when he started questioning it. By the end of the process, he was much more certain that it was biased, unhelpful and rather limited.

However, the way to deal with thoughts is not just to interrogate them until they beg for mercy. The point of the exercise is to give you more freedom, more options and more ways of seeing things. The 'questioning' stage is just one step on the road to expanding your thinking.

Step 2: Expanding your thinking

In this stage, the aim is to find *three alternative thoughts* about the situation. The main point is that they are different from the thought that you were having before, that's all. However, if you have just gone through the questioning stage, you will probably already have some thoughts that are more interesting and will give you more choices than your initial thought.

Let's follow Pete through this phase:

I need to get three alternatives. What are my top three things to remember from questioning? I think they are:

1. *I don't know what will happen in the future – I may surprise myself.*
2. *Thinking about failure all the time is depressing and gets me nowhere.*
3. *It could be a lot worse. There is plenty of time to keep trying.*

I don't think that having these thoughts will magically

make me lose weight, but it's a lot better than sitting around moping about being a failure. I know that I have got options and I'm not going to limit myself by presuming that I will always fail.

Developing your skills in dealing with automatic thoughts

There is one main thing that you need to do now to move forward – and that is to practise. Like any skill that is worth having, changing your thinking will take a bit of time and effort. However, it is a skill that you will be able to use for the rest of your life. After a while, it will become easy and automatic. It applies in all sorts of situations, not just weight management. Any time you spend developing this skill will be time well spent.

The basic steps of changing your thinking will be familiar to you now. They are:

1. Spot a difficult situation.
2. Follow the feeling.
3. Pinpoint the thought, explain and summarise exactly what the issue is.
4. Question the thought, expand your thinking and keep going until you have three alternative views.

You need to start doing this regularly, day by day, and writing things down in your notebook. It is absolutely necessary to write everything down at this stage. It's quite impossible for anyone to hold a thought, ten questions, all of the answers to those questions and three alternative thoughts in their head at once!

However, this doesn't mean that you will be making notes for the rest of your life. After a while this will become a new mental 'habit' and you will easily be able to spot thoughts and see interesting new perspectives. However, everyone has to start slowly and carefully, doing the exercises by the book, before real skill can emerge.

It can actually be very useful to notice your thoughts about the process of changing thoughts! Look at your thinking right now. Are you being optimistic or are you thinking, 'I'll never get the hang of this'? Are you having thoughts about yourself – perhaps 'I'm rubbish at this kind of thing' or 'I'm really smart! I'm sure I don't need to practise.' All of these are useful thoughts to spot, question and expand. You don't have to use thoughts about weight – any thought will help you develop your skills.

Some examples

Here are a couple of examples that might help you. To save space, we have just organised the 'questioning and expanding' around three questions:

1. How true is this thought? Is it biased?
2. How helpful is this thought?
3. What are other ways of thinking about the situation?

Look hard at how the thought is dealt with each time. This will give you ideas for your own practice.

> *I don't want to spend my life counting calories or going to the gym every day.*

How true is this thought? Is it biased?

> *Well I know that counting calories and attending the gym is one option, but I don't think they are for me. It might work for some people, but I need to find something else.*

How helpful is this thought?

> *Well, it's not a very hopeful thought – so it's not very helpful. Just because one approach wouldn't work doesn't mean none of them will.*

What are other ways of thinking about the situation?

> *There are many different approaches to managing weight and the key is to find what works for me, so I can follow it in the long term.*

What about this thought?

> *'Losing weight will be awful – I'll be hungry/miserable/ deprived all of the time.'*

How true is this thought? Is it biased?

Well, it's certainly true that most of the diets I've been on have resulted in me feeling deprived and hungry, but then most of them were pretty strange diets. I did feel physically hungry sometimes but mostly I just craved foods I told myself I couldn't have. Maybe if I didn't ban foods it might be different.

How helpful is this thought?

Maybe this thought is trying to make sure I don't feel miserable again by going on another diet. But there are definitely disadvantages to thinking like this. I scare myself and make myself less likely to do something new. In fact, thinking like this is so depressing it makes me prefer not to think about weight at all. And one thing is for certain: I won't manage my weight and health if I avoid it.

What are other ways of thinking about the situation?

First, this approach to managing weight may be different – this time I won't ban foods and I will be concentrating on being more active as well as eating differently. Secondly, thinking that it will be awful just makes me avoid thinking about it – and that will get me nowhere. Finally, maybe it's just time to try something out – just give it a go and see what happens – rather than trying to predict the future and scaring myself.

Now that you understand the basics of dealing with automatic thoughts, here are a couple of tips that can help.

Advanced tip number 1: Sometimes question thoughts that are obviously true

This may seem like odd advice. Clearly, there are some thoughts that are not worth challenging – like the fact that Paris is the capital of France. (This seems to be true and unbiased, fairly helpful if you are a tourist, and alternative views of the situation are not likely to get us far!) However, it is important to remember that thoughts can do a very good job of convincing us that they are true. Take, for example, this person who is in the process of pinpointing a thought:

> *Well, I think the main thought is I can't bear to stick to a diet. I just hate feeling deprived of food, it just gives me cravings the whole time. Of course, it would help if my husband were a little more helpful about the whole process. But I think the main thought is: 'I will hate any weight-management programme because I will feel deprived.'*

This is a good piece of pinpointing – the person here has really worked out what she is afraid of when she thinks about a new attempt to manage weight. However, she may have also missed a thought that may be important to explore in more detail. She seemed to think it was 'obvious' that things would be easier if her husband helped more. This may or may not be true.

When a person realises thoughts like these are just thoughts, not necessarily the truth, questioning them can be very valuable. It can really help us to see things we are missing or that we would usually need another person to point out to us.

Advanced tip number 2: If you are getting stuck, make sure that you are questioning a thought and not a feeling

Questioning and expanding a thought can sometimes be difficult if the thought is something like 'I'm sad' or 'I'm so anxious'. In this case, what you have found is actually a *feeling*.

The basic difference is this:

- A feeling is an emotion or sensation that can usually be put in one word.
- A thought is a statement about how things are, or how they should be, a prediction, a view of the world, an idea about a person, the world, the future, what should or should not happen. . . There are an infinite number of thoughts, but they can very seldom be expressed in a single word once they have been pinpointed.

If you have found a feeling, that is fine, and you obviously have good emotional awareness, but you need to work out the thought associated with it. For example, what are you sad about? What has gone wrong? What do you fear is happening? Perhaps what you find is: 'I'm so sad, I really can't cope with this situation.' In this case, 'sad' is the feeling and 'I can't cope' is the thought.

Keep practising. . .

Becoming a 'thoughts expert' only comes down to a few steps: spot upsetting situations and issues, pinpoint the thoughts, and question and expand your thinking. Appendix I has the whole process for quick reference. As we go through the book we will occasionally suggest that you do a 'thoughts check' when you look at certain issues.

As you go through your daily life, keep looking for automatic thoughts about weight. They can be found everywhere! If you look at a shop selling your favourite food or catch a glimpse of your body in a changing-room mirror, you will find them there. You will be able to see them when you are trying a weight-management programme and when things get difficult and aren't going to plan. As you become more aware of how your mind works this will give you more freedom to change. Self-awareness always brings more freedom. This is the topic of the next chapter.

CHAPTER SUMMARY

- We are thinking all of the time – about ourselves, other people, the future, what should and should not happen. . .
- We tend to think that our thoughts are true. However, a lot of the time they are untrue or unhelpful.
- Unhelpful thoughts often come up near strong emotions or stuck habits. It's useful to learn to spot these thoughts.
- Once a thought has been found, questioning it and expanding on it can give a person more options about how they feel and what they do.

3

Self-awareness

Self-awareness is a good thing, but to be honest, I've got it already. I know there isn't really a link between what I eat and what I weigh.

I really don't see where self-awareness is going to get me. Surely it would be better if I could just be getting on with a diet and exercise plan?

The last two chapters have been about thoughts and motivation. By now you may well be thinking, 'When are we going to start actually making some changes?'

When a person wants to manage their weight, it's natural to want to 'get on with it'. 'Diet' books often offer a 'plan' that you can start straight away, but for many people this approach often doesn't work long-term. This book offers an alternative – the skills you need to manage your weight for the long term. It shows the way to change habits, and to make those changes stick.

This approach is to change 'from the inside out'. This means starting off having a clear understanding of your own eating and activity habits and how they link to weight change. Once you're clear about which habits to focus on change can begin. Most other methods try to change 'from the outside in'– that is, they take a plan and try to 'drop' it full-scale into a person's life, but the chances are it won't fit and may not focus on the habits most relevant to you.

There will be more about how to change from the inside out in chapter 6. This chapter, however, is about understanding your usual daily habits and how they are linked with weight change.

How to understand your day-to-day habits

Spending money is a daily habit just like eating and drinking. Thinking about this analogy can help us think about weight. Imagine that you are keen to save money. You have something exciting that you want to do – go on a particular holiday, for example. However, this is going to cost money. You look at your income and it seems that there should be money to spare at the end of each month. However, this never seems to happen – there is no spare cash for your project. It looks as though your plans for saving – and your holiday – are never going to get off the ground. How would you fix this problem? How would you find out where the money was going?

If you were going to fix your saving problem, you would need to know exactly how much money was going in and out of your bank account. You could then work out how much you were spending and what you were spending it on. You might find that your loan repayments or house bills are more expensive than you thought. Or perhaps you are spending more than you thought on clothes, music or going out with friends. Of course, knowing this might not fix the problem straight away. However, you would still be able to decide how you could make changes.

In order to manage weight, it is essential to have the equivalent of a bank statement. You need to know, in detail, how much activity you are doing each week, how much food you are eating and how these are affected by various factors. Then, just as a person might need to 'balance' their income and their spending, you need to 'balance' your eating and activity if you are going to manage weight and improve health.

Some people might think this level of detail is too much. After all, most people have some idea of how much they eat. Although 'bank statements' may seem unnecessary to really understand our spending, it is helpful to have more information than our memories alone provide.

Consider:

1. What did you have for breakfast yesterday? And lunch? And dinner? What snacks did you have between meals?
2. And how many minutes did you spend walking?

Most people find it very hard to answer these questions with any accuracy.

Also, many people are baffled by how their eating habits lead to weight gain, particularly if they feel they don't over-consume excessively. This is when close noticing and monitoring of daily habits can be most helpful. Recognising that small changes in certain habits can impact on weight change and health over time is important.

Getting an accurate record of activity and eating

One of the challenges in managing weight is that we do not have an accurate record of eating and activity (like a bank statement) to help us to analyse the situation. However, we can make one. There are many different ways of doing this: keeping a written diary, dictating on to tape, taking photographs and/or using a mobile app. Whichever method you choose the important thing is to create a living fascinating record that includes feelings, thoughts, urges and all of the situations and habits that go with them.

Recording eating and activity is an active learning process. Whilst you are recording your habits, you will also be noticing your behaviour and developing self-awareness. Noticing what you are doing is often the first step in changing habits.

Imagine you're spending too much money every month so you decide to write down every penny spent. If you did this carefully, this is likely to reduce your spending because you notice each time money is used. This effect has been shown in many scientific studies – as soon as we become more aware of our behaviour, it tends to change. So, recording habits is a good way to gather information, but it is also the beginning of change.

Situations, moods and behaviour – how to record habits

So, what is the most helpful way to record daily habits?

To answer this question, it's a good idea to think about the purpose of recording and what it would be like to have a detailed understanding of our habits.

Kirsty has been recording her habits for about three weeks and is getting some very useful information.

There were some surprises when I started recording my eating. I knew a couple of things already – first, that my meals seemed pretty healthy (to me, at least), and second, that I did tend to eat a bit more when I was feeling low. I hadn't expected to find I ate more when I was in a good mood, though. When I was out with friends, I enjoyed myself, ate whatever I wanted and chose bigger portions and fattier foods.

I was right about my meals. They are healthy but I often eat large amounts. I also thought I ate more when I was low but it's actually when I'm stressed. I think I use it as a kind of reward for surviving busy times.

Snacks are a bit more of an issue than I had thought. There are always lots of biscuits at work but because I only have a couple with a cup of coffee I didn't think this was relevant. But keeping a food record has helped me notice how many coffees I have during the day and there-fore how many biscuits. On average I have four coffees a day, that's eight biscuits a day, and to be honest I don't even remember eating most of them. I definitely need to think again about how I manage this.

I've also noticed my exercise plans don't quite work out as I thought they did. Before I kept records I would have said I went to fitness classes two to three times a week and walked for at least an hour a day. But in reality I attend classes once or twice a week and probably walk about 20 minutes a day. It also helped me understand the reasons why I end up not being as active as I'd planned. When I was in a good mood, I might think, 'Life is too short for the gym' and see some friends instead. After a busy day at work, when I was stressed and tired, I just couldn't face it, so I'd curl up on the sofa instead with a glass of wine and some snacks.

My job is really sedentary too. I spend most of the day sat in front of a computer, usually drive to work and use the lift more times than I'd realised.

I wouldn't say recording my habits has been enjoyable and I've often felt like not doing it, but it has been really useful. It's helped me understand the things I do that were going under my radar, the things I was under- or over-estimating and what was linked to why I was doing these things. I now feel much clearer about where I need to make different plans.

When I first started keeping records I felt upset and frustrated with myself – 'I can't believe I eat that many biscuits – is it any wonder I'm so big?' – but these self-critical thoughts just made me feel worse and more likely to turn to comfort foods. So, I've been working really hard at noticing these thoughts for what they are. . . just really unhelpful.

Most people would agree that Kirsty is in a much better position now she knows these things – she is much more likely to make changes that will be effective. She got these results by recording just three things for activity and eating:

Situations – where she was, what she was doing, whom she was with.

Moods and physical feelings – what was going on with her emotions and body.

Behaviour – what she actually did, in detail.

These three things are the backbone of all recording.

A typical eating record

It is easiest to understand how to record eating and activity habits by seeing a good example of a record. This is a small section of an eating record written by Kirsty on a slightly boring Saturday when she was cleaning up and expecting visitors.

Situation and time	Mood, sensation	Eating
12.05 Between bits of housework and paying bills. On my own	Bored	Small tin of baked beans on two slices of brown toast. Low-fat spread
1.40 As above. Had just watched some TV for a break (bad TV)	Bored Irritated by TV	Three crackers, three tablespoons of houmous
2.40 Finished cleaning. House now officially ready for guests!	Pleased Relieved	1 cup of coffee, two chocolate biscuits

Although this is only a small piece of a record, it is already useful. It's clear Kirsty has healthy meals but snacks often. Further records would show whether this was linked with boredom, the day of the week (not at work), or the activity (cleaning up/housework). When Kirsty understands this, she will be better placed to think about making changes.

Later on in this chapter there are some specific ideas about recording activity and eating but, meanwhile, here are some general ideas about recording that may be helpful.

General principles for helpful recording

Recording situations

As you can see from Kirsty's record, it is not necessary to write down everything about a situation. A summary is enough but there are some things worth focusing on.

It's often important to record which other people are around – or if there are *no* other people around. Being busy or having nothing to do, where you are – at home, in a restaurant or late-night store – are also important. The time of day is often relevant, or if there are other situations that seem to be important to your habits, then record these as needed.

Recording moods and sensations

As it's helpful to know how emotions affect habits (they almost always do) include these in your records, e.g. sad, happy, stressed, angry, disgusted. Also include physical sensations like food cravings, hunger, fullness, tiredness or feeling bloated. These are not really emotions but may have important effects on habits.

It's not uncommon for people to become very unaware of physical sensations (such as hunger or fullness or thirst) particularly if they've dieted for many years and/or become used to ignoring the body's physical needs due perhaps to time pressure or busy work schedules.

Increasing awareness of physical sensations such as hunger is important, but before starting to include this in your records it's helpful to understand the difference between the various types of hunger.

Different Types of Hunger

We often use the term 'hunger' to describe a variety of different sensations. Making the distinction between these different types of hunger is critical because they need to be managed differently.

UNDERSTANDING PHYSICAL HUNGER

Physical hunger usually occurs a few hours after a meal, will often build gradually over time and goes away quite quickly once you've eaten enough. Some of the signs might include:

- Hunger pangs or a rumbling feeling in the stomach
- Emptiness
- Irritability
- Light-headedness
- Difficulty concentrating

When we eat in response to physical hunger we usually feel satisfied afterwards and it's a pleasant experience. Physical hunger is a normal sensation which we feel at various points throughout the day (unless we graze frequently) and is the body's way of prompting us to seek food. There is a common belief that in order to manage weight we will need to put up with feeling very (physically) hungry all of the time. This shouldn't be necessary and just requires careful management (*see later chapters*).

UNDERSTANDING EMOTIONAL HUNGER

Emotional hunger feels very different to physical hunger. It can happen at any time of the day; its onset can be quite quick and it's often unrelated to how long it's been since you last ate. So emotional hunger can happen right after a large meal even when you are already full. The sensation is usually in the mouth, head, chest or heart area and *not* the stomach and is sometimes called head hunger or food cravings. Eating in response to emotional hunger may not result in feeling satisfied afterwards and is commonly associated with regret or shame. Usually emotional hunger is linked to feelings or sensations such as boredom, anxiety, sadness, loneliness, procrastination, pain, stress or tiredness, and becoming more aware of these can be very helpful. Positive emotions such as happiness or joy can also lead to emotional overeating.

Be aware that your surroundings can also have an important effect on your desire or urge to eat. So, the sight and smell of food can increase 'hunger' or desire for food and explains why food advertising, cookery programmes or passing by the bakery can have such an impact on food cravings. Being aware of this is important during record keeping.

So, before you have a meal or snack or have a desire to eat, pause and ask yourself:

'What type of hunger do I have?'

Physical or emotional? If you're struggling to work this out ask yourself:

'Are the sensations in my stomach or my head?'

'How long is it since I last ate?'

'What other feelings do I have?'

If it's emotional hunger see if you can identify what feelings, emotions or sensations you are experiencing alongside the emotional hunger. What is your body really asking you for? For example, sleep or relaxation? Comfort?

If it's physical hunger try gathering more information about how hungry you are. You can do this using the scale below.

Ask yourself: 'Where am I on the hunger scale?' Record the number in your records.

The hunger and fullness scale is a useful way of improving your awareness of the levels of physical hunger and how this links to when and what you eat. As with all self-awareness though, make sure you are building the intent of learning about your habits rather than being critical about yourself.

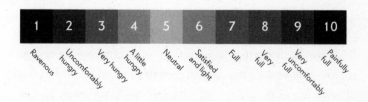

We'll explain more about how to manage these different types of hunger in later chapters, but the first step is to really tune in to the different types of hunger you're experiencing, what might be linked with emotional hunger and/or your levels of physical hunger before eating.

Fullness levels are also worth noting, so record your levels of fullness after eating using the same hunger and fullness scale.

As well as pausing before a meal or snack to rate levels of physical hunger, also try to build in a pause halfway through eating and at the end of the meal to check levels of hunger and fullness.

Recording behaviour

The main tip here is to provide enough detail. It's really important to describe any behaviour clearly, so that another person who did not know the situation would have a chance of understanding it properly. For example, different people mean different things by 'going for a swim'. For some people this may be a few leisurely lengths while chatting to a friend, and for others it's continuous intense swimming.

Amounts Count

Another important consideration in recording behaviour is that *Amounts Count*. Small amounts of food or physical activity can make a big difference in the long term. Earlier, we saw how changes in standard portion sizes can make a big difference to food intake over time. So, it's important to record amounts.

It is also important to record drinks. Alcoholic drinks and non-diet soft/fizzy drinks can contribute large amounts of excess calories and sugar, so it's worth noticing when and how much of these are consumed. Likewise, with the amount of sugar added to tea, coffee and other drinks. This process can also help people understand how much or how little fluid is being drunk. It may be, for example, that inadequate fluid and dehydration is part of the explanation for tiredness and fatigue which is sometimes managed with sugary snacks rather than addressing the real need of adequate fluid intake.

Recording amounts doesn't have to mean weighing food or timing activities to the nearest second. It's about finding a balance between recording amounts precisely and going 'over the top' with exact recording.

Recording activity

Two recording forms – one for activity, and one for eating – are included in Appendix I, pages 364 and 367, and you can photocopy these for your own use. This section explains how to use the activity form to get as much useful information as possible.

It's easiest to show this using the example of Kirsty's average work day. Have a look at it – it will mainly explain itself, but we will go through it in more detail below.

Time	Situation	Moods or sensations	Activity
03.00		Asleep	
04.00			
05.00			
06.00			
07.00	Shower, breakfast	Tired!	Stand for 20 mins – in shower and having breakfast
08.00	Car	”	Sitting
09.00	At my desk	Busy, concentrating	”
10.00	”	”	”
11.00	Tea break, chatting	More relaxed	Stand for 10 mins
12.00	At my desk	Busy	Sitting
13.00	Lunch break, gone out	Relaxed, happy	Walk for 15 mins, climb 3 flights of stairs
14.00	At my desk	Busy, stressed	Sitting

15.00	"	"	"
16.00	"	"	"
17.00	Car	Tired, headache	"
18.00	Got home! TV	Relaxed, happy	"
19.00	Making dinner	Irritated	Standing for 30 mins
20.00	TV/chatting, not going to gym	Distracted	Sitting
21.00	"	"	"
22.00	"	"	"
23.00	"	"	"
24.00		Asleep	
01.00		"	
02.00		"	

Important automatic thoughts:	I'm exhausted, I need to rest

Kirsty's record is quite simple. It just records situations, moods and behaviour. However, it's useful to look at how she has recorded her activity. Most people who work in an office sit down most of the day. (Of course, Kirsty stood up and walked around a bit whilst she was working, but it didn't amount to much, so she just recorded it as 'sitting'.) However, there is a big difference between sitting and standing. It may not seem like much of a difference, but anyone who tries standing up for a whole working day – eight hours – will certainly know the difference! The same goes for walking. Try standing for an hour and then try walking briskly for an hour – there's a huge difference. And this translates into a big difference in the amount of energy a person burns. So, when recording activity, it's helpful to record at least these five levels:

1. Sitting down or lying down
2. Standing
3. Walking
4. Moderate activity – walking briskly, doing house-work or gardening
5. More vigorous exercise – jogging or exercising in the gym

If you want to record more than this, you can. For example, it can be a good idea to record the number of flights of stairs you have climbed or how vigorous your activity was – for example, a slow walk or a brisk walk.

Kirsty's recording tells her a lot. It's clear that when she's at work, she doesn't move much. In fact, she is not really able to because her job keeps her sitting at the computer. Increasing activity would need to occur in her breaks, during the evening or while travelling to work. Also, there doesn't seem to be much of a relationship between her mood and her activity, as she was more active when relaxed (lunch) and irritated (dinner). She avoided going to the gym by getting distracted in front of the TV – this is something that she could work on.

At the bottom of the form, there are two extra sections. There is a space to write any important automatic thoughts that come up during the day and a section for a pedometer or step-counter reading. There will be more about pedometers and step counters in the next chapter.

It's best to record activity as you go through the day but if this really isn't possible try and write at the end of the day. It only took Kirsty five minutes to record her day's activity.

Recording eating

Recording eating is a little different from recording activity, as it is easier to record what is eaten rather than what happens in each hour. The recording forms that we recommend for eating are a little different and again can be found in Appendix I. Otherwise, the recording is very similar – it just covers situations, moods and behaviour. This is a sample of Kirsty's eating record:

Situation and time	Moods or sensations	Eating
06.45 Breakfast	Tired, not very hungry	Big bowl of cereal, skimmed milk Big glass of fruit juice
09.00 Making coffee at work	Tired, frustrated	Two biscuits, coffee with milk and sugar
10.30 Another coffee (break from computer work, quick chat with colleagues)	More awake Hunger 5	Two biscuits, coffee with milk and sugar
13.00 Lunch with friends	Relaxed, happy Pre-lunch hunger 3 Fullness 7/8	Chicken baguette (about 10 inches) with mayo and salad. Packet of crisps. Yoghurt, small pot

		Another coffee (milk and 2 tsp sugar) with a biscuit
15.00 Mid-afternoon break. Walk to canteen	Stressed, rushed Hunger 5	Medium-sized flapjack
16.30 Final coffee of the day	Stressed Hunger 5	Two biscuits
17.45 Just got home	Relieved Headache Hunger 2/3	Slice of toast with peanut butter. Two big teaspoons of peanut butter snacked from the jar
18.30 Dinner in front of the TV alone	Irritated Hunger pre meal 4 Fullness 8/9	Pasta in a tomato sauce (big plate). Parmesan on top. Half a baguette of garlic bread
20.00 Watching TV	Distracted Hunger 5	Glass of wine. Slice of toast with peanut butter

Important automatic thoughts:	I'm really busy. I deserve some biscuits

Again, looking at this record gives Kirsty useful information, even though it only covers a day. We can see her meals are fairly healthy, although fruit and vegetable intake is low, some portions may be a little out of balance and high-calorie snacks are frequent. Of course, she would not eat exactly the same every day, and it would be better to look at a couple of weeks of records to get a clear picture. However, it is clear making some changes to snacking habits could improve the healthiness of her behaviours.

There are not many really clear links between Kirsty's moods and her eating. However, the thought that she recorded is one clue. 'I'm really stressed. I deserve a biscuit' is a classic 'permission-giving' thought – combine this thinking with work stress, and Kirsty will eat a lot more. . .

How to do it

Hopefully, it is now clear why recording is useful, and roughly how it can be done. However, it can be hard to do. Like all other changes in behaviour, doing it in the middle of a busy life presents challenges. This section contains some ideas that can make things easier.

Which method to use

You can use the blank forms in Appendix I, pages 364–8, but you can collect information using the method that suits you best. Some people prefer to use a small notebook, which is compact and easy to carry, or a phone app, such as My Fitness Pal or Carbs and Cals, which are user friendly and use food photographs to guide portion selection. Remember, this book is about self-management so choose the approach that works best for you – for some ideas on how to use your smartphone, see the appendices.

When to do it

Many people have busy days and it is not easy to see when they could record food and activity. It can be particularly hard if someone wants to keep this process private. However, these difficulties can be overcome. Recording behaviour really takes very little time, maybe ten minutes a day, and there are few people who could not find this time.

Ideally record behaviour as you go along so it is as accurate as possible. Recording the next day is probably too inaccurate to be worthwhile due to our difficulties remembering our habits.

How long to do it for

It is not necessary to record behaviour forever. Remember the point is to provide you with useful information about your behaviour and build the habits of self-awareness and self-observation. So, recording needs to be done for a while and then stopped. It is often useful to go back to it, though, if you get 'stuck' in managing weight or if you start to regain weight and are unsure why.

You can choose whether you are going to record both eating and activity at the same time or do one at a time. It is up to you – this is a self-management approach and you can make the decision. However, it is important that you cover both eating *and* activity. If you just record one of the two, it is like looking at a bank statement and only analysing the money going in, not the money going out. This approach would be quite useless in understanding your money situation and the same is true with weight. Likewise, it's not just understanding how much money is coming in and out but also those factors that trigger overspending or earning less.

Common problems and difficulties

In our clinical experience, some people do find recording difficult. They are often reluctant to do it. Here are some positive ideas to help out with the most common problems.

'I really don't have the time to do this'

This is a common concern. Many people have busy lives and do not want to add anything else to their schedules. However, it is useful to 'question and expand' the thought. Is this really true that you don't have time? In fact, there is almost no one who does not have a spare ten minutes in their day. Most people, if they are really honest, and really want to, can find the time.

When a person thinks 'I don't have the time', this is often not what is really going on. In fact, what they actually mean is 'This is not a priority for me at the moment' or 'I am not willing to give up any time to do this'.

If a person seriously wants to find ten minutes in their day, they will do it. If they are not willing to, that is their choice – and it is a perfectly valid one.

If you are having difficulties seeing recording as a priority, then we suggest that you go back and look at the 'reasons' you found in chapter 1. See if looking at these makes any difference to your priorities. On the other hand, if you just don't think recording will help, keep reading – we will come to this soon.

Forgetting to keep records can also be challenging, particularly at the beginning of the process, so thinking through ideas of what might help can be important. Consider using phone reminders or alarms, keeping records to hand and visible, or linking recording to other routine activities.

'I can't bear it, I'm just too ashamed'

Some people feel deep shame about their eating or being active at their current size and this can make recording habits challenging. Seeing these habits written down in great detail may increase the sense of shame so it's not surprising monitoring may be avoided.

Although shame can be a difficult issue, it's important to explore it because it tends to keep people stuck in their current situation. Shame often leads to avoidance – either in thinking about, talking about or acting on a situation and this usually makes things worse.

So how do you deal differently with this?

1. It can be helpful to recognise the difference between guilt and shame. Take the example of eating half a packet of biscuits sitting in front of the TV late at night. Commonly there are two types of reactions to this experience.

    Reaction 1:
    'I wish I hadn't done that – it really wasn't part of the plan, but I've had a stressful day and I feel so tired'

    Reaction 2:
    'I'm such an idiot, is it any wonder I'm this big. Why, oh why, do I always do this, I'm so weak'

    In the first reaction, guilt about the action of eating too many biscuits is being expressed – they regret the *behaviour* – wished they hadn't done it as it wasn't part of their plan. In the second they believe the behaviour [eating lots of biscuits] says something really negative about them *as a person* – weak and stupid. This is shame and it's never helpful in making changes to habits – it has a really unhelpful impact on mood and motivation and increases the chances of repeating the behaviour [eating biscuits] when the same situation arises again [stressed or tired]. Try and notice these self-critical thoughts and use the skills developed from chapter 2 to question whether they are true, biased or helpful.

2. Be kinder to yourself. As you record your habits be on the lookout for self-critical thoughts popping into your head. As you become more self-aware you may notice you make harsh judgements about your habits. So, increasing awareness needs to go hand in hand with not judging yourself harshly for your behaviours. Try and think how you would talk to a friend or someone you are close to if they told you they ate in the same way. What would you say to them? Remember no one chose to be born with a brain that encourages food seeking or a metabolism that favours weight gain. You may have coped with difficult situations or feelings using food as a comfort – but this doesn't mean you're a weak person or a failure – it means you were doing the best you could with the skills and resources available to you at the time. With new skills and a deeper understanding of what affects your habits you can really begin to change from the inside out.

'It won't help me' or 'I've done it before, and it didn't work'

The first step here is to see these problems as thoughts, not realities, and to use your 'question and expand' skills. Whilst many people have kept food diaries in the past, most people have not tried recording in the way described in this chapter. Remember, the purpose of recording is to work out where you need to focus change but it isn't a magic cure.

If you do not think that recording will help, or you think you're already aware of your habits, that is fine – you may be right but it's worth doing an experiment to see if you are.

There are three easy steps:

1. Write down everything you ate last week and the amount of time that you were active. Write down lots of detail and exact quantities. Don't leave anything out.
2. Now monitor your eating and activity for this week. Use the forms and do it well.
3. Compare the two – your guesses for one week and your recordings for the next week.

If your recording is really no more accurate than your guesses and really doesn't add any understanding at all, then you can skip the rest of this chapter.

'I really don't want to mess about with forms and records. It's not really my kind of thing'

Writing things down on paper every day is certainly not everybody's idea of fun and it's human nature to want to limit recording.

However, imagine you are a running coach. A person comes to you saying they plan to be a brilliant 10,000-metre runner. They want to do it well and win prizes. However, after the first couple of weeks you realise that they aren't doing enough training. You confront them with this. They say to you, 'Yeah, but I find this training thing a bit boring. You see, I'm a bit of a free spirit. I'm not the kind of person who likes rules or schedules.'

What would you say to them? It would probably be something like, 'Well, I understand that it's hard work and it may be a bit new and a bit of a shock to you. However, if you want the results, we know this is the best way to do it.'

'What if someone finds the record or sees me making it?'

It's understandable to want to keep this information private and you can choose a method you think will offer the greatest privacy. Phone apps may be helpful in this situation as they are less likely to be stumbled across by someone else, your phone can be password protected and you could be using your phone for any number of reasons.

How to make sense of it all

If you do the recording well, you will have lots of valuable information that will help you identify key habits. You may begin to get ideas about things you can change. Sometimes though it's a bit harder to make sense of everything, so here are a few ideas to help.

Look for the Big Things

A helpful way to analyse your records is to concentrate on each part one at a time – behaviour, moods and situations. Start by focusing on the right-hand column where you recorded eating or activity and focus on the Big Things – the things you eat in large amounts (either all at once, or over a long period) and times when you are inactive (sitting or lying down) for a long period. These are usually important for weight management, as they are the times when we take in a lot of energy but may not burn it off.

As well as Big Things, it can be useful to look for Broken Plans. We may have good intentions about eating and activity but sometimes things go wrong. Although it's tempting to avoid thinking about these times, they are really important moments that hold useful information to help us change. They often show the situations and moods in which our plans go wrong and give us an idea about how to do something about them. It will be most interesting to see the moods and situations that go with Broken Plans.

Finally, it is important to look at Overall Amounts. Even if your eating seems reasonably healthy this has to be balanced against how active you are.

Moods and physical sensations

Next look at the 'Moods and Sensations' column. Sometimes people notice they are more angry, for example, or stressed, than they previously thought. It is sometimes not clear what to do about this, but at other times it can be really helpful to stop and think about how to meet these needs. Maybe you need to think of practical ways of managing stress – yoga, meditation, activity, or more help and support.

When looking at moods and sensations, try to see if any regularly turn up next to Big Things or Broken Plans. For example, a person might find a day full of boredom tends to go hand in hand with frequent snacking. Feeling tired might go along with breaking plans for exercise. These are fairly obvious examples – see if you can find your own.

Finally, have a look at the thoughts that go with these moods or sensations. This will often complete a very useful picture of what's happening with Big Things or Broken Plans.

Situations – look at times and places

The same applies to situations – look for situations that go with Big Things and Broken Plans. Look hard at particular times and places – for example, if you're on your own or in company. Overeating late at night is a common experience. Look particularly at the situations in which you seem to be most vulnerable.

The timing of eating and activity can be important. Waiting too long between meals may result in becoming extremely hungry, which increases the chances of eating large amounts or choosing different foods than planned. Look at your records and see where the largest 'gaps' between meals are, and how much you eat afterwards. You may also be more likely to break activity or food plans at particular times or in particular situations. For example, you may be able to exercise in the evenings, but only on the way home from work, rather than going out again after returning. These are all important pieces of information. Try to notice your own patterns.

Useful information

Everything that you pick up from your records about Big Things, Broken Plans or Overall Amounts of food or activity is useful information and you can make notes under each of these headings. It is the starting place for changing from the inside out.

However, by making all of this effort you have done more than just collect information. You have developed the skills that you need to understand your own habits. You can use these skills and techniques at any time in the future. If you get stuck in the process of managing weight – a really common experience – returning to monitoring your habits for a while can be very helpful. It will often give you the information you need to get back on track.

Now you have done the important foundation work for managing weight – looking at motivation and thinking patterns, and developing self-awareness.

Next we will look at how to make real changes.

CHAPTER SUMMARY

- This book shows you how to change from the inside out – that is, how to understand your current habits and begin to make changes.
- To do this, you need a detailed understanding of your eating and activity habits.
- The best way to do this well is to record them, and to include important information like situations and moods.
- Analysing your records can provide important clues about your habits.
- Building self-awareness is an important skill in managing weight.
- Remember to try to be kind to yourself as you monitor your habits and use the skills from chapter 2 to explore self-critical thoughts.

PART TWO

MAKING CHANGES

4

Changing physical activity

To say I hated sport at school would be an understatement. The humiliation of never being picked for a team, the cruel comments from other people in my class and the horror of having to get undressed and showered with everyone else. . . Now whenever I think it would be a good idea to start going to the gym, all these memories come flooding back.

Perhaps when you think of physical activity this is the sort of thing that comes to mind. Unfortunately, negative experiences of activity are common for many people, and not just in children or adults who struggle to control their weight. Early experiences can have a lasting impact on how you feel about being more active in adulthood. Or perhaps you used to enjoy being active or playing sport but haven't done so for a while, so knowing where to start can be quite daunting? Or perhaps you've never been a particularly active person? It can be helpful to consider what kind of experiences you have had and your ideas about activity in case these might be stopping you from being more active today.

So, what does activity mean to you? Does it mean:

- Taking up a sport
- Having to be competitive
- Being totally exhausted at the end
- Doing it but hating every minute
- Spending hours in the gym every day
- Wearing tight, uncomfortable clothing
- Feeling self-conscious and vulnerable
- Feeling you're just no good at sports
- Being surrounded by people who are very fit and slim and don't understand your situation

These are very common thoughts and experiences, but it doesn't need to be this way. Being more active can mean:

- Reducing time spent being inactive/sitting
- Changing the way you might get from one place to the next
- Spending 10 to 15 minutes being active a couple of times a week
- Doing something you enjoy and at which you have developed a skill
- Having fun, with being active becoming just a by-product of what you are enjoying
- Feeling stronger as you get fitter

There is a common belief that for activity to help with weight management it needs to be structured exercise like going swimming or jogging, attending exercise classes or working out at the gym. These options are good ones for some people but for others these types of activities would be a struggle.

Interestingly, activities that are sometimes thought of as not making much of a difference when trying to manage weight, like walking more, are particularly helpful ways of increasing overall activity. They are also less likely to be linked with some of the negative feelings described above. So, it's very important to broaden what we think of as 'physical activity' to include walking, gardening and vigorous housework, etc.

The key to becoming and remaining more active is to choose activities that are likely to be enjoyable and/or give us a sense of achievement, rather than things that are done solely to lose weight. This chapter aims to help you identify activities that might work for you in the long term, and what might get in the way.

Is changing physical activity really that important?

There is good evidence that activity gives us:

- An improved sense of wellbeing – the 'feel-good' factor – that many people describe during and after activity

- A sense of achievement
- Clearer thinking and memory
- Reduced anxiety and stress
- Improved mood
- Improved sleep quality
- Improved strength, mobility and flexibility
- A reduced chance of developing chronic health problems such as heart disease, high blood pressure, high cholesterol, colon cancer, breast cancer, diabetes and depression
- For people with an existing chronic health problem, improvements in how well the condition is controlled
- A maintenance of muscle during weight loss (so helping to keep metabolism as high as possible and burning as much energy as possible)
- Help with managing pain

All of these benefits are important, although some will be more relevant to you than others. It can be difficult to be enthusiastic about the importance of activity when the benefits (like reduced risk of heart disease) might not be experienced for another ten to twenty years. Instead of thinking about the long-term benefits it can be more helpful to notice the immediate benefits – improved mood, feeling less stressed and anxious, and a sense of achievement.

Lisa's story shows the pleasure that taking time out and including more activity can achieve. Walking was not an activity that she had thought of as exercise or something that would make much difference to her weight, but when her doctor advised her that this could be the way forward she thought she might as well give it a go. The difficulty was finding the time to be active with a busy job and a young family. In the end she decided to walk to the local park – which was about 10 minutes from the office – during her lunch hour. On some days she'd sit and have her sandwiches there, maybe walk round the park if she felt like it and then head back to the office. She would feel so much more refreshed when she was back at her desk and, although she'd been worried about taking this time out, she felt she worked better for having had a break.

What Lisa really began to enjoy was the time on her own, something she never really experienced at home any more – she had time to think about things and clear her head. What the walking was doing for her weight almost stopped mattering; it just made her feel so much better.

The enjoyment that activity can bring is often forgotten, especially if you have negative memories of being active.

The role of activity in keeping weight off

Activity can help with weight loss when used alongside changes to what we eat, but it is more difficult to manage weight with activity alone. However, being active certainly has an important role to play and is also the best predictor of who keeps weight off and who regains it, so building physical activity into your life at this stage is extremely beneficial. Also, as physical activity has a powerful anti-depressant effect, it can help with weight loss indirectly – if we are active we are more likely to feel motivated, and if our mood is more buoyant we are better equipped to deal with challenges when things get tough, and to make healthier choices.

So how can we get more active?

Knowing what not to do

As already mentioned, unfortunately a person's previous experiences with activity and exercise often leave them with unhelpful ideas about how to become active. Also, there is a lot of talk in the media about what does and doesn't work when it comes to physical activity. Noticing if you have any of the thoughts or beliefs that follow can help you identify what might get in the way of becoming more active.

'Right, now I'm going to become really active' – too much, too soon

Being determined and enthusiastic about being more active is important. However, this can mean that you set very tough targets for yourself. Trying to do too much too soon can result in giving up completely. It's usually helpful to check that the changes you choose are realistic not just in the first few weeks when changes are high priority but also over the long term. (Check out chapter 6 for more details of how to make SMART changes.) Increases in activity need to be built up gradually, particularly if you have been fairly inactive for some time. Doing too much too soon is also likely to result in physical discomfort or even injury and this can be very off-putting.

'I really need to "feel the burn" if this is going to work'

There is a common belief that for activity to be beneficial it needs to be very hard work and to hurt – no pain, no gain. This is simply not true; activity doesn't need to hurt to be extremely effective. Indeed, pushing too hard and 'going for the burn', particularly if you're not fit at the time, can risk injuries to muscles and joints as well as put you off activity on a regular basis. A little muscle soreness the day following activity is to be expected when you first start being more active, but if you're in pain while exercising you should stop. Working at a pace that is comfortable for you offers all the benefits to health, fitness and weight and is a more enjoyable experience, so one you'll want to continue.

How do you know when you're working at a good pace but not overdoing it? A good rule of thumb is the 'talk test'. If you're breathing harder than usual but you can still manage to talk without gasping for air then you're likely to be working at a moderate intensity, a level that will give you health benefits and is more sustainable. More of this later in the chapter.

'A couple of weeks of activity will change my body shape and size'

Hoping for too much too quickly is very understandable but can lead to frustration and a feeling that being more active just isn't working. It is human nature to want visible results overnight, but it's important to try and make sure you don't have unrealistic expectations of what can be achieved.

Activity is unlikely to make a big difference to weight in the first few weeks unless large amounts of it are being done, and for most people this is neither realistic nor wise. But this doesn't mean that activity isn't important. As well as its many other benefits, it has a vital role in helping to keep weight off.

It's worth knowing what to expect from activity and what it might achieve before starting out with any changes:

- You can expect the feel-good benefits and the sense of achievement to be immediate. There will also be immediate internal changes in your body too (for example, improved blood sugar and hormone regulation) but you probably won't notice these at first.
- After 4 weeks strength, stamina and general fitness will improve if you have consistently increased your activity.
- Changes to body shape and weight will usually start to be seen after 10–12 weeks of regular increased activity.

One of the reasons why activity is advised in combination

with changes to eating is because, as mentioned above, activity changes on their own will result in fairly slow progress with weight management and shape change. It is very difficult to lose more than about ½ lb every two weeks or so by only changing activity, particularly if you haven't been active for a while and you're building up fitness slowly. Changing only activity habits can be the way forward for some people, as long as they can keep motivated to continue. But focusing on the immediate benefits of activity, the 'feel-good' factor and the achievement of doing regular activity, may help more than thinking only of how much weight has been lost or calories burned.

'Exercise makes me hungrier'

I really don't know why I bother exercising. It never helps me lose weight. Swimming is my favourite activity, but when I come out of the pool I'm just so hungry I find it almost impossible to resist getting something from the vending machine. What's the point of going swimming if it's just going to cause me to eat more?

Exercise can feel like it increases appetite. However, research has shown that activity has very little effect on physical hunger, except when done very intensely for long periods, similar to the levels of an athlete.

So, what can the explanation be for this common belief? One suggestion has been that although increased activity doesn't result in a physical trigger to eat more (unless we are exercising at very high levels) it might change the way food choices are thought about. So, it might be something along the lines of 'I've just swum thirty lengths so I deserve a chocolate bar.' Sometimes activity can be used as a way of giving ourselves permission to eat something as a reward. Of course, eating a chocolate bar is fine so long as it's part of your overall plan. However, it can interfere with weight loss if it happens frequently, and also if you begin to associate an activity with a food reward. Also, if few other food changes have occurred or the plan for losing weight focuses only on changing physical activity, rather than a combination of food and activity, there will be problems. Another challenge is certain foods and drinks are promoted as being necessary if we are exercising, such as energy bars and drinks. These usually contain a lot of calories (for 'energy' read 'calories') and are not necessary unless we are exercising at a very high level. So, it is important to be aware of how our thoughts about food choices can sometimes change as activity increases.

It might also be that what we believe to be physical hunger turns out to be food cravings. Chapter 7 gives more details of how to work out the difference between these two feelings and how to cope with cravings.

Sometimes the explanation for strong feelings of physical hunger after activity can be quite practical and might be to do with the timing of meals and snacks. It may be that the activity is done before work, so breakfast might be a bit later than usual, or on the way home from work, so the evening meal is delayed, and hunger levels would therefore naturally be higher than if no activity had been done. Planning ahead can be particularly helpful in these situations. Taking a healthy snack – something like a banana or yoghurt – that can be eaten straight after the activity can take the edge off hunger until the next meal. This avoids having to grab whatever food is available at the time and this can be really important at times when hunger levels are high. The hungrier you are, the more difficult it can be to make the healthier choice. It can also be helpful to think about having a small healthy snack about an hour *before* activity to help prevent hunger during and after activity. However, how the body responds to food before activity can vary quite a bit from person to person, so if you find that even a small snack close to being active can leave you feeling a bit sick or sluggish it is probably best to skip this.

'Activity burns a lot of calories'

Activity *can* burn lots of calories, but to do so it must be quite intense and quite frequent. This level of activity is well beyond what most people can manage.

How many calories are burned by being more active will vary from one person to the next, depending on their weight and gender. As a general rule, half an hour of moderate activity will use up about 200–250 calories, depending on the type of activity. This may seem like a lot of effort for not many calories worked off but of course the importance of activity in helping to manage weight goes far beyond how many calories are used up.

People often believe they are burning off more calories through activity than they really are. This probably doesn't matter unless they use it as part of their decision about food choices. It is common for there to be a mismatch between what someone believes they are working off and what they then decide to eat, for example: 'Well, I've just jogged for thirty minutes so that will have burned off an extra slice of pizza.' Jogging for 30 minutes will burn off about 300 calories, whereas a large slice of pizza will be about 400 calories. If mismatches like this occur regularly it can interfere with managing weight.

Linda's story illustrates how thinking can change as activity increases, and this can result in unknowingly eating more:

I usually drove to work but had recently started to walk and was pleased with how well I was doing. Not once had I taken the car in the last month. So I was shocked when I found out my weight had actually increased. My usual reaction to this would have been to give up completely, but I was so determined this time to make things work that I stopped and made myself really think through what had been happening. It took me some time, but I worked out I'd been rewarding myself with extra food for all the effort I'd put into walking. Without really realising it little thoughts had popped into my head like, 'You've been really good with the walking, so it'll be fine to have an extra biscuit.' They were really brief thoughts, but I reacted to them and ate more than usual. Finding different ways of rewarding myself was essential.

Knowing what to do

We've looked in detail at some unhelpful approaches to changing activity and taking time to think these through can often be enough for changes to begin to take place. This next section moves on to considering what might be helpful and how much to aim for.

How much activity makes a difference?

The recommended amount of physical activity for improving health in adults is 150 minutes per week of moderate-intensity activity or 75 minutes a week of vigorous activity. Moderate activity is when we are a little bit warmer, have a slightly increased heart rate and are breathing a bit faster – a good way to tell if activity is moderate is if you have enough breath to talk but would struggle to sing! For vigorous activity, heart rate would be higher, you would start to sweat after a few minutes, and breathing rate would increase to a level where you would struggle to talk. How much we need to move to be active at a moderate or vigorous level will vary a great deal from person to person – for example, the average person's level of moderate activity will be very different to that of a professional sportsperson. It can also vary a lot over our lifetime – we may have had a higher level of fitness when we were younger and could do more, so we need to be realistic about where we are starting from now. It is important to understand what moderate means for you to avoid doing too much too soon. As well as moving more, it's recommended that we include some sort of

139

strength training or weight-bearing activity twice a week, too. This could include housework, carrying shopping, arm raises with filled water bottles at home when watching TV, yoga where we build strength using our own body weight, as well as the more obvious lifting weights at a gym. Finally, regardless of how active someone is we should also try not to sit for long periods without a little bit of movement.

These recommendations can be broken down in all sorts of ways, so the 150 minutes of moderate activity could be 50 minutes three times a week or about 20 minutes every day or something in between. For people who are more used to being active and enjoy working out at a vigorous level the total of 75 minutes vigorous-intensity activity can be broken down in a similar way or combined with moderate activity. Any movement, however brief, counts.

The good news!

This much activity can sound quite overwhelming. Many people struggle to do this much, so if you are one of them please don't worry – the good news is that if you are doing less than 150 minutes, any increase can actually make a big difference to your health. You don't need to do the full 150 minutes to gain many of the benefits and we will offer some ideas on how to increase the amount you are doing. The important thing is to build up slowly and find something that suits you. For example, the latest evidence advises that an additional 10 minutes of brisk walking (or similar moderate-intensity activity) on most days of the week would lead to significant benefits in the long term for most of us, but if you are starting from doing nothing, adding in just a couple of minutes each day could make a big difference, too.

Assessing your current level of activity

Working out how active you are at the moment is the first step in deciding what, if any, changes you want to make to physical activity. Keeping records of activity as described in chapter 3, pages 105–9 is a very helpful way to work out how much you are doing at the moment, so it would be useful to write down any periods of moderate- or vigorous-intensity activity you do during a typical week and if you do any weight-bearing exercise.

Many people also find working towards a daily step-count target is helpful, and using 10,000 steps a day has commonly been used in the past as a way of defining if someone is active or not. Although it is now thought to be more accurate to measure the amount of time we are active, and at what level (moderate or vigorous), step counts are still a useful and clear measure of activity. Most smartphones have an app that automatically measures your steps, so if you have a smartphone this can be a helpful way of checking. If you are not sure how to do this you can search online for 'measuring steps' and the type of phone you have. There are also lots of wearable devices that track all sorts of activity including steps (e.g. Fitbit, Garmin, Jawbone and Apple Watch), as well as more basic devices such as pedometers that are cheap to buy online or in sport shops.

Once you have an idea about how much activity you are doing at the moment it's time to start thinking about what you might like to add in – more of this later.

What might be stopping you from being more active?

If you've assessed how active you are and feel this might be something you want to begin changing it can be helpful to check through anything that might get in the way of you making these changes, applying what you learned in chapter 2.

Listed below are some of the common reasons that people struggle with being more active. Some of these may be relevant to you, others may not, but the process of thinking through possible barriers to increasing activity is often useful. Do any of the following sound familiar?

- A negative experience of activity
- Not feeling confident in your ability to be active
- Lack of time
- Finding it expensive
- Finding it boring
- Not feeling like it, low motivation
- Disappointment with the 'results'
- Fear of injury or damaging health
- Don't feel safe
- Worried what other people might think of you/ body image

If you feel the barriers listed opposite are holding you back, here are some ideas that may help you to discover some solutions that are specific to you and your lifestyle. Lots of these ideas cross over, so for example your solution for not having enough time might also be the same solution as for not feeling like it.

Negative experiences of activity

It can be helpful to think through why the experience was negative. Was it to do with what you had to wear or where you had to get changed? Or did you feel you just weren't good enough at the activity? It may be none of these reasons, but this gives an idea of the kind of questions to think about.

Once you've worked out what puts you off, it's possible to start thinking through other options. So, if the competitiveness of some activities is not something you enjoy, you might consider alternatives such as walking, gardening, dancing, water aerobics or yoga. Broadening what is thought of as activity can be useful here. If you feel self-conscious doing some activities on your own, could you do something with others? Would being active with the support of a friend or family member be helpful? Can you think of an activity that would help you feel less under pressure, such as walking?

Not feeling confident in your ability to be active

This is often connected to difficult experiences of activity that may have knocked your confidence. It is all too easy to think that if you're not good at one or two activities then you're just no good at exercise in general. Of course, this isn't the case. Only a small number of people are naturally good at sport. The majority need lots of coaching and practice – something that may not always be encouraged if the skill isn't naturally there. We also want to stress that when we talk about physical activity we mean any sort of movement in the broadest sense, so you do not need to go anywhere near a sports field or do anything that involves Lycra! – unless you want to, of course.

Again, think through options that don't involve 'being good' at something or having particular skills but which have all the same benefits for health, weight and wellbeing.

Lack of time

This is a common barrier to being more active. Moving activity up the priority list in a busy life can be difficult, but it is possible. It isn't necessary to be active all in one go – it can be divided up during the day into five- or ten-minute sessions that can be easier to fit in. In fact, this can be even more helpful than doing all your activity in one chunk as it breaks up the amount of time you are inactive.

Combining activity with socialising can also be an option if being active with others appeals to you – a day with the family in the park, joining a local walking club or trying a dance class are just a few of the many possibilities. You might also want to think through how you can build activity into your day to *save* you time. For example, it might be quicker to walk between bus stops on busy routes than to take the bus, or to walk up escalators. In cities, many people find that cycling is the fastest way to get around.

Finding an option that is convenient is important. If you decide to go swimming a couple of times a week in the evening but find that once you get home it's too tempting to just stay there, consider other times that may be more helpful or a pool nearer work. Would taking your swimming kit to work and then going to the pool on the way home make it easier? Or would a swim at lunchtime or first thing in the morning be a better option? Also, there are lots of great activity classes available free online that can be done at home at a time that is convenient for you.

If lack of time feels like a barrier, it can also be really important to schedule activity into your diary so that it happens and doesn't get squeezed out by all the other things you need to do. Fitting activity into a busy life does have the added bonus of actually helping with the hassles of a hectic schedule by reducing stress and improving mood and sleeping habits.

Finding it expensive

Joining a gym or taking up a new sport can be expensive, particularly if lots of equipment is needed. However, it isn't necessary to choose these options to gain all the benefits of activity. There are a number of activities that cost nothing but provide all the same benefits for your health and weight. Walking is one of the cheapest activities, with the only equipment needed being a good pair of shoes. And again, the internet offers lots of options for a range of classes that can be done at home.

Finding it boring

This can be the case if you've chosen an activity you're not really interested in or don't enjoy very much. Being active with others can be helpful here, as can being active outside if that appeals to you. Building additional enjoyment into an activity can also change it completely, for example listening to music, podcasts or audiobooks, or watching TV shows at the gym. As we are creatures of habit this can also help us build activity into our routine – we could decide to only watch our favourite TV show when we are at the gym or listen to the next chapter of a book when walking. That way our brain begins to associate the pleasurable activity with the physical activity. Of course, it is possible to start out doing an activity you enjoy but then to lose interest after a while. If you feel this might happen to you it can be helpful to choose a variety of activities to keep up your interest and motivation.

Not feeling like it

Quite often we might find it really difficult to actually get started with being active, despite making plans. This is a really common experience – when asked, even many top elite athletes report that they often don't feel like training before they start but enjoy it once they begin! Most people, once they do get started, and particularly after they finish, usually feel much better. It can be helpful to remind ourselves that it is normal not to feel like exercising or being active and that to an extent we just have to ignore these feelings and get on with our plans. To help with this, it's important to make activity as easy and pleasurable as we can for ourselves. Deciding to just take mini steps can also help, for example if you plan on going jogging when you get home from work but don't feel like it, you could choose to just put on your trainers and active clothing. Once these are on you could decide to just go for a walk around the block. Chances are once you have followed each of these stages you might just find yourself jogging anyway. Practically, setting up how you can make it as easy as possible to be active is important, for example putting on your 'active' clothes on as soon as you get home from work or leave the office, or leaving them out the night before if you are going to be active in the morning.

Related to not feeling like it is also not feeling motivated. Not feeling motivated is often linked to either not feeling confident about doing something or not feeling it is important, or both! If you think your low motivation might be linked to lack of confidence, hopefully this chapter will offer some ideas for activity that you might be able to try. It might also help with finding reasons why activity is important in a general sense, but if you still feel that activity is not important for you we would suggest revisiting your notes from chapter 1 on motivation. By connecting your reasons for wanting to change, and your response to the Five Years exercise to physical activity, you might be able to make the link between activity and how it will bring you closer to your values.

Disappointment with the 'results'

As we've already mentioned, expecting increased activity to bring rapid results either with weight change or differences in body shape will probably lead to disappointment. Check that your expectations are realistic at the outset. Focusing on the achievement of being more active rather than on the physical changes in body shape that activity will produce is often a more positive approach. You might also like to make a note of how you feel after each time you are active and track whether this changes. Improvements in mood during, and particularly after, activity are often quite immediate and a result that shouldn't be underestimated.

Fear of injury or damaging health

This is an understandable concern, particularly if you haven't been active for a while or have a health condition. If you are worried, and particularly if you have a health problem, it is wise to consult your doctor before starting. However, it's worth bearing in mind that almost all health conditions that are not in an acute phase (haven't just happened) tend to improve with gentle increases in physical activity. For most people who have some level of mobility, walking is a great option. Remember that beginning slowly and building up gradually is important; listen to your body and make sure that you are staying within the moderate range of activity (talk not sing) rather that working too hard when you start. For people for whom walking isn't an option there are chair-based physical activity options that can be just as effective and can be done at home or in groups. If you need more information about this your doctor or consultant will be able to help.

Not feeling safe

If you live in a neighbourhood where you wouldn't feel safe being active on your own it can be useful to look for options where you can exercise with others by joining a class or group, or by trying out different options at home. For example, if you would like to walk more, free or low-cost local walking groups are often available to join. For jogging/running there is the 'Parkrun', who organise free runs around the world (parkrun.org.uk). They are open to everyone and encourage people to take part at their own pace, including walking or using a wheelchair.

It can also be helpful to reflect upon what not feeling safe means for you and if there are ways of overcoming this. For example, starting out by being active during daylight, being aware of your surroundings, not wearing headphones, letting people know where you are, exercising where there are other people around, etc.

Worried what other people might think of you/ body image

Many people feel self-conscious when they start being more active, regardless of their body size. If you also feel self-conscious because of your weight this can add an extra level of concern. Again, choosing an activity where you might feel less self-conscious, such as walking, or starting an activity with a friend can help. In the longer run, as you become more confident about your ability to be active, you might feel more able to challenge these concerns and take part in a wider range of activities. It can also be helpful to remember that it is not uncommon to feel self-conscious in this way. Most people are more worried about how they look when they first start being active rather than noticing their surroundings or the people around them. As we become more familiar with an activity and new surroundings we usually become a little less self-conscious, so sticking with it for at least a couple of sessions is also a good idea.

Which activities are helpful?

Any activity that involves moving the body more than usual will be beneficial to health and weight. Some of these approaches may surprise you. . .

Cutting down on sedentary activities

Look first at how long you spend doing inactive hobbies like watching TV or sitting at the computer. Some people spend hours like this as a way of relaxing. Of course, this is fine if other ways of being more active are also part of their lifestyle. But too much screen time has been linked to problems with weight.

Again, changing this behaviour is not about making extreme changes – it isn't necessary to ban yourself from ever turning on the TV again. But think through how long you spend sitting in front of a screen and then consider ways of spending less time doing this. Setting an alarm to stand up and move around every 45–60 minutes, even if only for a minute or two, can really help.

The other problem with television watching is that it is often linked with eating high-calorie snack foods, and food cravings are common while watching favourite programmes. TV adverts and cookery programmes showing various tempting high-calorie foods don't really help with this either. And often whatever we eat while sitting in front of a screen isn't really fully recognised or enjoyed. Many people have experienced a bowl of food 'disappearing' whilst they were watching TV. So, cutting back on time spent watching TV or doing other sedentary activities not only helps increase overall activity but also makes food changes easier.

Increasing lifestyle activities

Unfortunately, in today's society it's very easy to be inactive. Lifts and cars mean we don't need to walk much and washing machines, dishwashers and vacuum cleaners have made many household chores much easier than they were thirty or forty years ago. The weekly shop can be delivered to the door without having to move away from the computer screen, and many of us have jobs that require sitting for long periods of time. These changes in how active we need to be in our daily lives have made a big difference to how inactive many of us are – our grandparents would probably have been much more active than us without going anywhere near a gym. Of course, there is no need to give up useful time-saving advances. However, it does mean we have to think about how we can incorporate more activity into everyday life.

Building more activity into the way we live our lives can be a really useful way of increasing overall activity. It may not seem as though doing more gardening or washing the kitchen floor vigorously to music will make much difference to weight, but all of these changes added together really can be helpful.

Here are some changes that people have used as a way of increasing their lifestyle activity:

- Taking several trips upstairs rather than piling things on the stairs for one trip later
- Doing own house-cleaning and gardening
- Taking activity breaks during commercials
- Getting up to change channels rather than using a remote or Alexa
- Taking your dog for walks rather than just letting them loose in the garden

- Parking at the furthest end of the car park and walking to the shops
- Taking the stairs rather than the lift
- Taking activity breaks every hour during the working day
- Taking a short walk during lunch break
- Using a bus timetable phone app to play 'beat the bus' – if your bus isn't due for 10 minutes could you walk to the next stop?
- Taking a daily 'wonder photo' of something that catches your eye when out walking
- Walking to the local shops rather than driving
- Standing when on the phone
- Marching on the spot when brushing your teeth

Think through some of your day-to-day habits and see whether there is any way you could 'choose the active option'. You might also like to consider using some sort of wearable device to track your activity, which can be very rewarding. More on these below.

A word about walking

It can certainly be helpful to think about increasing how much we walk. You can use amount of time walked at a moderate level and/or a step count. Even if we are nowhere near reaching 10,000 steps it can be great to set a target to work towards, particularly if we can also try to incorporate some brisker walking at a moderate level.

Even small changes can make a big difference, as **Kirsty** found:

> When I was first given a pedometer, I didn't have a clue what it was for or how to use it. But it was so easy. If someone had asked me before I did this whether I was an active person I think I would have said I was as active as most people I knew. But wearing the pedometer really brought it home to me how inactive I was. On most days I found it hard to clock up more than 3,500 steps, so I was definitely classed as inactive. And when I really thought about my activity, it wasn't surprising. I drove to work and would drive round for ages trying to find the parking spot closest to my building. I sat at a desk all day and always took the lift. At the end of the day I'd drive home and watch TV all evening, feeling completely exhausted.
>
> But using the pedometer and knowing what I needed to aim for was really helpful and motivating. I started with the plan of increasing my steps by 1000 each day, so I could reach about 4500 steps on most days. I started with a few small changes but was really surprised to see what a difference they made to the number of steps taken.

If you would like to increase your walking like Kirsty did, you can do this by measuring how long you are active for, at what level and by using a step counter or tracker of some sort. To use step counting as a way of increasing activity, make a note of the number of steps walked at the end of each day and then after a week work out your average over the week – many wearable devices will do this for you. Once you have an idea of how many steps you do in an average day you can work towards increasing this. We would suggest increasing your steps by about 500 or 1000 a day at first for a few weeks, noticing how you feel and then perhaps increasing again if you feel ready to. There are no hard and fast rules and it is up to you to work out what is most likely to suit you. You can also search for walking programmes online, based on your current activity level, or could consider joining a local walking group. Some people might want to build up to 10,000 steps a day or more but for others this isn't going to be realistic. Whatever increases you make, keeping it up in the long term is of great benefit. As well as being a useful way of keeping track, monitoring changes in activity can be very motivating. Wearable devices and apps also have the advantage of being able to do much more than just count steps. For example, some can also measure heart rate, distance travelled, flights of stairs. They can also set goals, give prompt reminders to move, increase goals as we become more active, and send rewarding messages when we reach a target. Lots of research has shown measuring devices, including very simple pedometer step counters, can be a real help in increasing activity, so it might be worth considering investing in some sort of activity-measuring device, however basic.

You can also search for walking programmes online, based on your current activity level.

Increasing aerobic activity

Adding aerobic activity to your more active lifestyle will make your heart stronger and more efficient as well as helping with weight management. Jogging, cycling, swimming, dancing, racquet sports like tennis or squash, and rowing are all examples of aerobic activities. Aerobic activity should be done at your moderate level, particularly when starting out.

It's important to begin by establishing a routine. In the first few weeks or months, the focus needs to be on getting used to a regular pattern of activity and working out which days and times are going to be best for you. The first time you do your exercise you may manage, say, 10 minutes and then the same again at the second session in the week. You may not feel that this is much and may be tempted to really push yourself at the next session, but be careful about trying to do too much too soon. Simply maintaining your routine (how often you are active) needs to be the main focus in the early stages. Then, as it becomes more established, you can build on how long you are active for.

Warming up and cooling down at the start and the end of aerobic activity to prevent injuries are vital to help prepare and protect our bodies. A quick online search for 'warming up' and 'cooling down' exercises will identify plenty of guided videos to help you with this.

Changing activity habits is not easy and it takes time to

establish a new routine and to feel comfortable about it. It is often necessary to experiment with what will work for you and how best to fit activity into your lifestyle. Remember, if one approach doesn't work that doesn't mean you can't 'do' exercise, it just means you need to try an alternative way of being more active.

How does it apply to you?

Having read about the benefits of activity and how you might address some of the unhelpful approaches and barriers to being more active, it's useful to stop and think through in detail how all of this applies to you. The following chart will help you to do this.

What are the benefits of activity for me?

_____

_____

_____

_____

_____

_____

_____

_____

What's stopping me being more active?

_____

_____

_____

_____

What would I need to change to be more active?

_____

_____

_____

_____

Which activities might work well for me?

_____

_____

_____

_____

Changing activity habits takes time, as we need to establish new habits and to feel comfortable with them. It can also help to remember that increasing activity is the quickest and most effective change we can make to improve our overall health.

CHAPTER SUMMARY

- Assess your usual activity levels by keeping records and/or using a step counter. Both of these will also help keep a track of changes to activity.

- As you plan ways of being more active it can be useful to consider the following questions: Do you find it helpful to exercise alone or with other people?

  Do you prefer to be active outdoors, at home or in the gym?

  How much money do you want to spend on being more active?

  What is the most convenient time of the day to be more active?

- Start slowly and set goals that are realistic. For example, if you've decided to walk more, adding a few more minutes a day will make a difference. It doesn't matter where you start from, so long as you build up from this point and keep going.

- Cutting down on sedentary activities and increasing lifestyle activities first can help build up fitness levels before starting on aerobic activities. And if you are already quite active but do have long periods of sitting, consider how you can break these up.

- Choose activities that you enjoy and feel comfortable with. Activities that make you feel self-conscious or vulnerable are going to be hard to keep up.

- Be aware of how tempting it can be to reward increased activity with higher-calorie food.

- With aerobic activity, establish your routine first before you begin building on how long or how hard you are working.

- Check you have appropriate clothing and sports shoes. Drinking plenty of water routinely is essential to prevent dehydration. Over a day our bodies need about six to eight glasses of fluid. When we are active we need extra water, particularly if we sweat. Water is the healthiest choice and, unless you're doing very large amounts of activity, sports drinks aren't necessary. Try to take sips of water before and during activity and drink at least a couple of glasses of water afterwards.

- Boredom is one of the most common reasons people give up, so choose activities you get something positive from, whether that's a feeling of wellbeing or enjoyment from practising a skill. Doing a variety of different activities is also helpful.

- Focus on the achievement of being more active rather than the eventual results of the activity.
- Any amount of activity counts, however small, and helps to improve mental and physical wellbeing.

5

Changing eating habits

'If only I could find the right diet.'
'Dieting is pointless. It doesn't work.'

These are common views expressed by many people who are understandably frustrated by the process of trying to manage their health and weight. It's easy to see why these beliefs develop given how challenging it is to change eating habits, but unhelpful beliefs make the process harder and limit the chances of making and sustaining new habits.

So, the first section of this chapter explores the truth behind commonly held food and dieting beliefs and considers how these can impact on changing eating habits. It may be tempting to skip this section, particularly if you've tried to alter your eating habits before and feel you already have a good knowledge. However, thinking through your beliefs and attitudes to changing eating can be a helpful step in deciding the best way forward.

This chapter is not about providing you with lists of suggested food changes or eating plans – there are already a number of books on the market that do that job very well (and some that do it very badly) – but to try and put you in the best possible position to make a truly informed choice about which approach to changing your eating habits is likely to be the most helpful for you.

Information presented in this chapter is in line with current medical and dietetic research and practice at the time of going to print.

Unhelpful beliefs about changing eating habits

'If only I could find the right diet. . .'

There is a common belief that managing weight is solely dependent on finding the 'right' diet and once identified weight loss will be easy and effortless. It's not surprising this belief is so common given our diet culture and the amount of marketing from the diet industry. New diets regularly emerge promising to be THE solution for weight loss and dismissing other treatments as ineffective. This marketing is clever and convincing, particularly if you feel frustrated about your current situation.

However, to answer the question about whether there is a best diet for managing weight we need to move away from diet-industry marketing and celebrity opinion and look at what the science tells us. A number of high-quality studies have recently shown there isn't one best diet for managing weight but rather a number of evidence-based options (more about these later) that achieve similar results. We know people respond differently to the same approach, so what works well for one person may not help another. What we need science to help us understand are the specific reasons why some people respond to a particular approach much better than others. While we wait for research to provide more guidance on who is likely to do best with which treatment there are a number of practical areas to think through that may be helpful in choosing an eating plan for you.

1. THINK THROUGH THE CAUSES OF WEIGHT GAIN

As already discussed in chapter 3, increasing awareness of the habits linked with weight gain and what may be triggering certain behaviours is really important. The more you understand about your eating habits and what triggers certain behaviours the more likely you are to be able to focus on management of these particular challenges.

2. THINK THROUGH WHETHER A PARTICULAR PLAN ADDRESSES THE CHALLENGES YOU HAVE IDENTIFIED

This is the crucial part that is often forgotten. For example, if you snack on lots of sugary foods during the evening because you experience food cravings which you believe are triggered by fatigue and loneliness, a plan that only focuses on your knowledge of healthier snack options is unlikely to be particularly helpful. You need an approach that helps you deal differently with these cravings, which teaches skills and strategies for recognising and providing your body with what it really needs.

3. DOES THE PLAN FIT WITH YOUR FOOD TASTES AND PREFERENCES, YOUR DAILY ROUTINES AND RESPONSIBILITIES AND ANY HEALTH CONDITIONS YOU MAY HAVE?

So, although it isn't about searching for the one 'right' diet, it is about developing an understanding of which eating plan you feel more able to follow. It might be helpful to think through how an eating plan fits with your daily routines and health conditions and whether it provides the support and skills training for long-term habit change.

'Dieting is pointless. It doesn't work'

Frustration with changing eating habits is a very understandable outcome of struggling to manage weight and can lead people to believe it's all pointless.

But let's explore this belief in a bit more detail. First, what exactly do we mean by 'dieting'? If we are talking about the latest celebrity diet or quick-fix approach (e.g. alkaline diet, blood-type diet) then this type of 'dieting' probably is pointless; it's very unlikely to help you achieve long-term habit change and may even be detrimental to health. For these fad-type diets there is no science to support their effectiveness and they are best avoided. They also tend to encourage a dieting mentality where people may begin to feel shame around their food choices because they have been unable stick to the strict food-based rules.

However, in its original sense the term 'diet' just means the foods regularly eaten or your usual food intake, so everyone has a diet of some sort. When people say dieting is pointless what they often mean is that changing eating habits is hard to keep up.

So, the challenge is not about looking for an alternative to changing eating habits but understanding more about what helps people sustain changes to their eating (and activity). You can find out more about this in later chapters.

Only recently has 'maintenance' of changed behaviour been recognised as an important issue. Traditionally people have been encouraged to just think about losing weight. It now seems that thinking through whether the changes you choose for weight loss can be continued in the long term might be much more important than initially realised. The next chapter deals in more detail with making changes work.

The importance of developing healthy eating habits is about much more than its effect on weight. There are now a number of studies that show improving the quality of the diet can reduce the risk of ill health even if there isn't much change in weight. So healthy eating habits are important even when weight remains fairly stable.

'I go for just one night out and by the next morning I've gained 3lb'

A weight increase after a night out can be very disheartening and may lead people to abandon their efforts to develop new habits.

Usually, though, it's not the amount or type of food that has been eaten that leads to long-term weight gain but people's reactions to eating more than they had planned. Many people have been on a night out, eaten and drunk more than planned and then thought, 'Well, I've blown it now, so I might as well really go overboard.'

Chapter 9 explains how to deal differently with these situations. The message here is to try and keep such events in perspective. It's useful to bear in mind that what is done on a day-to-day basis is more important than what is eaten or drunk on the odd night out, and even if there is a temporary increase in weight the next day this will often even itself out over the next few days as you return to your planned habit changes.

You may well be wondering how someone could see a 3lb weight increase if all they had done was have a beer and a curry. Body weight is not just a measure of body fat but of all the components within the body – the bone, muscle, liver, kidneys and fluid. Rapid rises in weight will most likely be due to increases in fluid that will resolve in time; women commonly retain fluid around menstruation, for example. (Under no circumstances should fluid intake be restricted as this will simply result in dehydration and have no effect on body fat.)

So, it is important to recognise that *what the scales tell you doesn't always mean what you think it does*. A person's weight goes up and down quite naturally during the day and from one day to the next for all sorts of reasons, including hormonal and fluid changes, bowel changes and the type of food and drink consumed.

For this reason, many people find weighing themselves

every day too confusing, although others find it helps keep them on track. It's difficult not to react negatively if you see a rapid rise in numbers and if this sounds like you, it may well be helpful to weigh less regularly and work on responding differently to the scale readings

'Salad is good for you, chocolate is bad'

Thinking about foods as either 'good' or 'bad' is not a helpful long-term approach to changing habits. Salad is certainly part of a healthy eating pattern, but chocolate can be too. Labelling foods with moral words such as 'good' or 'bad' or 'naughty' or 'nice' is common in the media and in popular weight-loss diets – so common in fact that it can be a challenge to stop. However, it's important to think through what effect this habit can have on your eating and the way you feel about yourself.

 Believing a certain kind of food is 'naughty' tends to make us want to eat it more but to feel bad or ashamed for doing so. Not only does this tend to remove our enjoyment of the food, but it can lead to the 'Well, I've blown it now so I might as well just continue' effect. The opposite can be true for food we think of as good for us. How many times have you heard someone say, 'I really don't like it, but I know it's good for me so I'm going to eat it'? This belief about 'good' food tends to make it less appealing and result in people feeling they 'should' eat it. As we saw in chapter 1, 'shoulds' do not seem to work for long-term motivation. Of course, some foods are healthier than others and can be eaten in larger amounts and more often. However, the overall habit of labelling is still not helpful.

It is far better to consider food for what it really is. So chocolate is a high-calorie food that can be included sometimes, and salad is a healthy food that can be (if you like it) included regularly. The important point is that *all* foods can be part of a healthy way of eating.

Working towards developing a more positive attitude to all foods can have long-term benefits. If you do think of certain types of food as 'bad', it is important to try and remove these labels and give yourself permission to eat these foods (*see chapter 2 for more details of changing thinking*). Successfully removing labels can help take away shame and ultimately improve your enjoyment of eating.

'As long as everything I buy is fat-free or low sugar, weight will drop off'

Foods labelled fat-free are often believed to be calorie-free but changing to fat-free products alone may not lead to the weight loss you expect.

There are two main reasons for this. The first is that fat-free, reduced-fat or low-fat products are not always the low-calorie choices we believe them to be. Second, there can be a tendency to increase the amount we eat because we think our food is calorie-free. Have you ever bought a packet of reduced-fat biscuits or cake, had one piece and then thought, 'Oh I'll just treat myself to another one. They are low fat, after all'?

Reading food labels is important for many manufactured foods – even those you may think will have little or no fat or sugar can sometimes be surprisingly high in 'hidden' fat or sugars. There is more on understanding food labels later in this chapter (page 207).

'If I skip a meal, that's a good start'

Sandra had been on and off various fad diets for most of her adult life. Over the years she had got into the habit of skipping meals during the day. When she first started to do this, it had seemed like a good way to lose weight. She regularly felt tired, a bit dizzy and irritable during the middle of the morning or late afternoon, but she got used to ignoring her body's hunger signals during the day and didn't feel the urge to eat until evening. Despite all this deprivation her weight had increased, and she struggled to understand why.

Although it seems logical to think avoiding eating during the day will lead to weight loss it is often linked with difficulty managing eating and weight. In Sandra's case by the time she got home she was so hungry that once she started eating she felt the urge to continue throughout the evening and she began to feel things were getting out of control. Allowing herself to become 'over hungry' had made it more difficult to make healthy food choices and manage portion sizes. She tended to think, 'Well, I've had a hard day and I've eaten nothing at all, so I deserve this.'

It's not uncommon for skipping meals and avoidance of eating for long periods to be linked to bingeing as shown

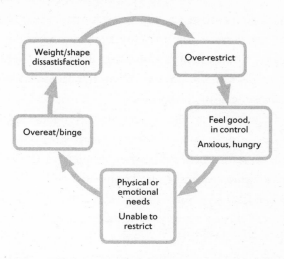

in the figure above. Although over-restriction of eating initially increases the sense of control, eventually some physical or emotional need such as feeling very hungry or anxiety or boredom will lead to eating. Foods may be eaten quickly and with little sense of satisfaction, followed by unhelpful thoughts and feelings and an increased determination to 'be good' (i.e. over-restrict) the next day.

Once Sandra had got used to the idea she needed to eat regularly during the day, to tune in to the signals her body was giving her and to respond to these in a helpful way, she felt more in charge during the evening. She was able to make the healthier choices she had planned and was less inclined to snack than previously. It took some practice, though, and she had to focus on understanding her hunger signals, but over time rather than avoiding hunger she began to respond to it in a helpful way.

There are no hard and fast rules about when to eat and it isn't necessary to stick to any rigid timetable for meals or snacks. You can eat at times that suit your lifestyle. For most people, though, it is wise to eat regularly, usually three times a day at least. Long periods without food will cause blood-sugar levels to fall and that can cause light-headedness, irritability and tiredness. Eating regularly keeps the blood-sugar level stable, preventing these unpleasant feelings, and makes healthier choices more likely.

More helpful beliefs

Here are some more positive – and accurate – alternatives to the unhelpful beliefs above:

- Finding a way of eating that suits you is only one part of understanding how best to manage your weight and health.
- Changing your eating habits is an important part of managing health and weight and means that realistic changes are more sustainable.
- Large increases in body fat do not occur overnight or after one night out.
- Weight will only be lost when energy from food consumed is less than energy used through activity. (This is not saying weight loss is simple!)
- Labelling foods with positive and negative tags

tends to lead to problematic attitudes to food and managing weight.
- Eating at regular intervals throughout the day is often helpful in managing weight.
- A good understanding of how to read food labels can be useful.

How weight is controlled

I just don't understand why I can't lose weight – I eat next to nothing and yet still gain weight.

This is a fairly common belief and in order to understand what's going on it can be helpful to learn more about how the body controls weight. This is a very complicated subject and involves a large number of systems in the body and complex interactions between hormones and various chemicals. It is true that energy balance is part of the explanation and it can be helpful to understand how this works.

The basics of energy balance

The control of weight is a balancing act between the amount of energy (calories) you take in from food and the amount you need to keep the body functioning at rest and when physically active. When you are 'in balance', the energy that you're eating equals that used by the body at rest and burnt off through activity, so your weight will remain the same. Only when your body goes 'out of balance' can you lose or gain weight.

Imagine a plastic container that can either shrink or expand depending on how much is stored inside it. At the top of the container is a water tap and at the bottom an outflow tap. When water is run into the container at the same rate as it flows out of the tap at the bottom, the container stays the same size. Only if less water goes into the container than is running out will it shrink (and vice versa).

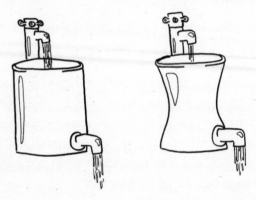

Now imagine the container is your body, the water flowing in is food and that flowing out is what is needed by your body for metabolism and activity. Body weight will only be lost when fewer calories from food flow in than go out as activity.

This is probably something you've heard many times before and it may not seem a particularly helpful explanation. It does tend to make weight loss sound simple – just eat less and exercise more – and we know that managing weight and health is not simple. What this explanation fails to highlight are the many complicated factors that influence what and why people eat and how active they are.

Nevertheless, understanding the basics of energy balance can be helpful when things don't go to plan. If weight loss isn't happening it may be either because too many calories are being eaten or not enough are being used up, or most likely a combination of both. This is a situation where recording eating and activity (*see chapter 3*) would be particularly beneficial in helping to pinpoint where changes may have slipped a little.

'My husband never puts on weight. It's not fair'

Sandra couldn't understand why she struggled so much with her weight. At work she would be the person with salad and cottage cheese on her plate while others piled on the chips and fried food. It was the same with her husband – he seemed to be able to eat whatever he liked and not put on an ounce. Life seemed very unfair.

Comparing your eating patterns to those of other people is understandable but isn't helpful for a variety of reasons. Let's take Sandra's situation again. She's 5 foot 3 inches and weighs 13 stone and she's just found out she has prediabetes and is keen to change some aspects of her lifestyle. At her current weight, Sandra's body will use up about 2000 calories each day. This means if she eats roughly this amount her weight will remain stable, any less and she'll lose and any more and she'll gain. Sandra would lose weight if she ate about 500 calories fewer than usual each day (i.e. 1500 calories a day). If you're interested in working out how much energy your body uses up each day, take a look at www.calculator.net/calorie-calculator.html where you can calculate your individual needs.

So, are there any differences between one person's body and another's in terms of their energy needs? There certainly are: it depends on how much someone weighs, the amount of muscle they have and how active they are. The higher their weight, muscle and activity, the more calories they will burn off each day. Sandra's husband is 15½ stone and his body uses up 2700 calories a day, so he can eat about 700 calories more than Sandra before he's at the point where he may gain weight. This is part of the explanation as to how he manages to eat more and not gain weight.

One of the key difficulties in Sandra comparing herself to other people is that in most instances she only gets a snapshot of what someone is eating throughout the day, even her husband. She may see what they eat at one meal and compare it to what she is eating, but this is often not an accurate reflection of the total amount eaten during the day. It is certainly not detailed enough to understand what their average intake is over a number of days or weeks. It's also very important to factor in how active someone is, and this can also be very difficult to judge accurately.

Probably the most important reason for it being best for Sandra not to compare herself with others is that it doesn't get her any further ahead in managing her own situation and will most likely just add to her frustration and lead her down the path of self-blame. What's more likely to be helpful is for her to focus on the factors that she does have some control over: her food and activity choices, and to try and work out through detailed record keeping what might be getting in the way of healthy eating and activity habits. As discussed in chapter 2, she also needs to work on avoiding self-critical thoughts about her current behaviours as this can be counterproductive.

What if weight loss has been going well and then suddenly it slows and eventually stops?

This is not uncommon and there are a number of possible explanations for why it happens. If large weight losses of say 15–20lb (7–9kg) have occurred then the slowing down may be due to the fall in metabolic rate that takes place with this amount of weight loss, and further adjustment of eating and/or activity may be needed. As weight falls there is loss of body fat and also some muscle, and it is the amount of muscle in the body that is a major determinant of metabolic rate. So, as you lose weight, you lose muscle, your metabolism drops, and your now smaller body needs less energy/fewer calories each day. Think of it as *not* having to carry round a bag weighing 15–20lb all day and how much less energy is needed as a consequence. Although this is an important effect it can be overcome with a few adjustments to eating (around 200 fewer calories per day) and an increase in activity.

If little weight loss has occurred before progress slows, the explanation is more likely to do with eating more than originally planned rather than a fall in metabolic rate. When we begin to make changes to eating habits we focus on and prioritise those changes, but over time this focus can begin to slip.

Jackie's experience of this is very typical. At first everything had gone well. She'd bought a steamer and changed how her food was cooked and had been really careful with the portions served. She enjoyed swimming, so she'd started going back to the local pool three times a week with a friend from work. She felt healthier, had more energy and the weight was coming off. But then on week six the number on the scale showed an increase of 1½lb (0.7kg). She just couldn't understand it, this was the first time since she started that her weight had increased, and it didn't make sense. 'What was the point of all that work?' she thought. 'I might just as well go back to what I was doing before and at least enjoy myself.'

Understandably, Jackie felt frustrated by the situation and reacted by believing the changes were no longer working and giving up on her new habits. But if she had paused and reflected on what was really happening things could have worked out differently. First, the weight increase was very small and if she had checked again a few days later it might have fallen. The key tool in this situation is self-awareness – to really check in with what has been happening with current habits and see if any changes or minor slips have occurred. It's important, though, to try and do this without the self-critical thoughts that have a tendency to pop up. In Jackie's case, without realising it she had become almost a little too confident about the weight loss and had tended to think: 'It's all going well so a little bit extra of this won't do any harm.' As this happened, her portion sizes and snacking had crept up. She did work this out by keeping detailed records of her eating behaviour and thinking through exactly what had happened.

Helpful approaches

We have looked in detail at some of the common food beliefs that are usually unhelpful when developing healthier eating habits. Taking time to think through unhelpful beliefs can often be enough for changes to begin to take place.

This next section moves on to consider more helpful approaches. Before considering specific approaches its often useful to see if anything can be learned from your past experience of dieting. (If you've never tried to change your eating habits before, please move on to the next section, A Review of Popular Diets, page 184.)

To learn from past dieting experience, it is important to take the time to think through which diets you've tried before and whether any of these were more or less successful. It may also help to consider other factors that influenced your ability to keep changes in place. See if **Sandra's** experience of dieting throws any light on this process.

OVERCOMING WEIGHT PROBLEMS

Which diet	When	Outcome	What interfered/Life events	Learned anything?
Cambridge diet	Age 23	Lost 3 stone in 3 months but quickly regained.	Sitting university exams. Snacking when stressed. Difficult to limit alcohol.	Eating in response to stress is a problem.
Weight Watchers	Age 27	Lost 4 stone over 1 year.	Motivation was fitting into wedding dress.	Group support helped keep me on track.
Weight Watchers (cont.)		Gradual regain over next 2 years.	Started new job after honeymoon and weight was less of a priority.	Lost my way a bit when new job started – was stressed and eating out was a regular part of the job.

180

Cabbage soup diet	Age 32	Lost 8lb in 1 week. Had regained 15lb 1 month later.	Struggling to adjust to life at home with a young child. A lot of snacking.	Felt very low about self when weight quickly returned.
Atkins diet	Age 33	Lost 7lb in 2 days. Regained 10lb within 2 weeks.	Gave up. Went to a wedding, friend's birthday and university reunion all in 1 week – disaster – dieting abandoned.	Really struggled to cope with the restriction of doing this one. Felt low.
Slimming World	Age 34	1 stone. Gradual regain when stopped going.	All was going well until I was offered a seat on a bus by a man who thought I was pregnant. I wasn't!	People say hurtful things!

It took Sandra a while to complete this chart (this is only a small section) and at the beginning she really couldn't see the point of doing it. But as she began to think through all her experiences, to record what had been happening at the same time and what she thought she'd learned, she began to recognise patterns to her dieting.

What would you conclude from her chart? You could say she had worked really hard and tried many different diets, she lost varying amounts of weight, but it was usually regained. So, you could conclude that nothing worked and changing her eating habits was pointless. However, looking in more detail gives more information.

Did any of the approaches seem to suit her better than others? Let's look in a bit more detail at her most successful attempt. This was achieved by attending Weight Watchers, where she lost 4 stone before her wedding day. However, it is not clear whether this success was due to the diet alone or to the very strong reason she had for making those changes. In reality it was most likely a combination of these factors. She believed regular support had helped keep her on track and had managed to sustain her eating changes for one year. This might be an approach to consider using again in the future. Likewise, with Slimming World she had been progressing well until a particularly hurtful comment had thrown her off track.

It's interesting to look at what seems unhelpful when she tried to change her eating habits.

Some diets just didn't suit her; the Atkins diet was too restrictive and she only managed a few days; similarly, the cabbage soup diet only lasted a week. Increased eating in response to stressful situations was mentioned a number of times and although Sandra had some awareness of this before completing the chart, taking the time to really think through her past experiences helped her see how her response to stress was interfering with long-term habit change.

She was now in a better position to consider which approaches to consider for the future, but more importantly was aware of the areas that she needed to focus on changing, i.e. coping with emotions and stress in other ways (*see chapter 7*) and ensuring she had good support to help her through some of the more challenging times.

Although your situation will be different from Sandra's, the principles are the same:

- Take time to think through what you've done before.
- Try to work out what helped and what didn't.
- Don't just focus on the 'type' of diet you chose but think through other areas of your life – they are often just as important.
- Try to work out what made it difficult to continue – feelings, situations, practical difficulties.

This process will hopefully help you to pinpoint not only the types of diets that are more likely to be helpful to you but also the factors that are helping and hindering you in making changes over the long term.

A review of popular diets

You only need to look at the bestseller book lists to know that there's no shortage of diets to choose from. However, the multi–million dollar question is: 'Which one will work best for me?' Although there's much more to managing your weight than finding the 'right' diet, working out which approaches are more likely to suit you is important, and there are likely to be ways of changing your eating patterns that will work better for you than others. And there are certainly diets that are better for your health – so which would you choose?

One of the most useful things to do first of all is to separate the extreme faddy diets from the more sensible approaches.

How to spot a fad diet

All of the below are warning signals that a diet is unlikely to be helpful. As a general rule of thumb if something sounds too good to be true then it most likely is.

- Any diet that promises weight loss will be quick, easy and painless – we know it isn't
- Diets that claim to remove body fat through 'detoxification'

- Diets that focus on just one or two foods – e.g. the grapefruit diet or the cabbage soup diet
- Lists of 'good' and 'bad' foods
- Whole food groups removed or very restricted
- Diets that include foods that 'melt away body fat' or 'raise metabolism'
- Diets that state foods have to be eaten in specific combinations
- Diets that suggest weight can be managed without changes to activity or lifestyle
- Rigid inflexible food choices and meal plans

Unfortunately, many of these diets are very cleverly marketed so they sound incredibly appealing. They seem to be the answer to people's prayers – a quick, easy, permanent solution. For most people, though, they offer little long-term hope of managing weight more effectively. Beware fad diets. No matter how tempting they may sound, avoid travelling down this much beaten but unhelpful track.

Safe and healthy diets

Reviewed below are some of the nutritionally sound dietary treatments that are considered to be safe and healthy. These may be helpful. But remember the diet itself does not hold the secret to success. It is only one piece of the jigsaw and to complete the picture it's essential to understand more about the factors that help or hinder you from putting these changes into practice.

LOW FAT

- **Examples:** *American Heart Association Low Fat, Low Cholesterol Cookbook*; *Healthy Eating: Low Fat Food*

- **What are they?** Most low-fat diets will suggest modest reductions in the amount of fat eaten, with an emphasis on substituting the animal sources of fat (fatty meats, butter, cheese) with healthier alternatives (fish, poultry, low-fat spread, reduced-fat cheeses). There are some very low-fat diets (e.g. *Eat More, Weigh Less*) that suggest severe reductions to fat intake that may be too restrictive for some people.

- **Do they work?** Restricting fat intake is one way of limiting energy (calorie) intake and there is evidence that low-fat eating is helpful in managing weight and, importantly, reducing the risk of various diseases that are linked to how we live our lives, such as heart disease. However, there is much more to eating well than just changing the type and amounts of fat eaten. It is the whole dietary pattern that is important – so although it's helpful to focus on fats, other aspects of the diet, such as vegetables, whole grains or sugary foods, need also to be considered.

- **Are they safe?** Yes, there's nothing to suggest that this approach is unsafe.

LOW GLYCAEMIC INDEX OR LOW-GI DIETS

- **Examples:** *The GI Diet*, *The Glycaemic Load Diet*, and *The Low GI Diet Revolution*
- **What are they?** Glycaemic index is a way of ranking carbohydrate foods (bread and cereals) according to their effect on blood-sugar level in the body. The theory is that foods which affect blood-sugar level quickly (high-GI foods) lead to a rapid return of hunger, whereas those that have a more steadying effect (low-GI foods) help us to feel fuller for longer. In other words, this is a diet that should help avoid large swings in blood-sugar and hunger levels. Refined starchy foods such as white bread, rice and cereals are high-GI foods, whereas whole-grain breads and pastas, barley and pulses are low-GI.
- **Do they work?** The jury is still out on just how helpful this type of diet is for managing weight, but it is a way of eating that contains many healthy foods (fruit, whole grains and pulses) that protect against heart disease and diabetes. Combining a low-glycaemic way of eating with changes to the amount and type of fat eaten may be a helpful way of managing weight and health for some people.
- **Are they safe?** Yes, there is nothing to suggest that this isn't a safe type of diet to follow.

COMMERCIAL WEIGHT-MANAGEMENT GROUPS

- **Examples:** *Weight Watchers*, *Slimming World*
- **What are they?** Lay groups often run by people who

have successfully managed their own weight using the commercial group they then go on to lead. They provide structure, education, skills and, very importantly, support from other people in similar situations. The support aspect of these groups is probably one of their most helpful features, although they don't suit everyone.

- **Do they work?** There is evidence for their effectiveness, with studies showing on average people achieve modest weight change of around 3–5 per cent less than their starting weight. As with all approaches to managing weight there is a variation in response, so this average figure includes those who respond very well and will lose more than the average, as well as those who for whom this approach doesn't suit and they will lose very little or may even gain weight. It's also important to consider the cost and time implications of commercial approaches.
- **Are they safe?** Yes. There is nothing to suggest that these approaches are unsafe.

MEAL REPLACEMENTS

- **Examples:** *SlimFast*, *Tesco Slim*
- **What are they?** Ready-portioned shakes, soups, bars or meals that can be used to replace two meals (and snacks) during the day with one healthy main meal of about 600–700 calories each day. Fruit, vegetables and increased intake of water are encouraged.
- **Do they work?** It's unclear how helpful this approach

is if the products are just bought off the shelf and used without any outside help or support. In settings where people have been supported this is a useful approach, with promising maintenance of weight loss particularly if one shake (or bar or soup) is used each day as part of the maintenance programme, Some meal-replacement companies do provide educational materials and internet support.

- **Are they safe?** Yes. There is nothing to suggest people are at risk from using this approach. Be aware though that some of the commercial meal-replacement approaches include a number of additional products in their ranges such as fat metabolisers, which have no evidence for their effectiveness, are often expensive and will not be helpful in managing weight and health long-term.

What about liquid formula diets?

- **Examples:** *Cambridge Weight Plan*, *Medifast*
- **What are they?** Usually liquid diets that replace all meals and snacks and severely restrict calorie intake to around 800 calories or fewer each day. They are used for only short periods of time and should not be used as the only form of treatment but in conjunction with counselling or medical treatment. Very low-calorie diets should not be undertaken lightly as there can be side effects and people need to be clinically monitored.

- **Do they work?** There is increasing evidence to suggest that properly supervised formula diets may be helpful in producing rapid initial weight loss, but this needs to be followed by a comprehensive maintenance programme that provides the support and skills needed to develop long-term healthy eating habits.
- **Are they safe?** There are side effects and risks and so it's important to consider these carefully with your doctor. Given there are some risks linked with formula diets this is not an approach suitable for people who are trying to lose a few pounds. Rather it is really for those with a higher BMI and health problems linked to their weight where the benefits of treatment outweigh possible risks.

What about low-carbohydrate diets?

These are popular diets and there has been much discussion in the media about whether a low-carbohydrate or low-fat diet is better for achieving weight loss and improving health. As we discussed earlier in the chapter, there isn't one dietary approach that has been scientifically shown to be superior, rather a range of options that achieve similar results.

- **Examples:** *Dr Atkins New Diet Revolution, The Carbohydrate Addict's Diet, Protein Power, Sugar Busters.*
- **What are they?** These diets substantially reduce carbohydrates, not only sugars and refined carbohydrates

like white bread and white pasta but some also restrict certain vegetables, fruits and whole grains. They may also encourage large amounts of protein foods (meat and cheese) and can be high in saturated fats.

- **Do they work?** There is research to suggest these diets are helpful in achieving weight loss for some people, but they have not been shown to be superior to other dietary treatments. Although some people may respond well to this type of approach, others may not, and they should not be considered superior to other dietary approaches discussed here.

- **Are they safe?** Most research that has investigated the safety of low-carbohydrate diets has not shown any harmful effects. However, there are still a number of uncertainties about how eating in this way could affect long-term health.

What about the Mediterranean Diet?

- **Examples:** Mediterranean programme and recipes: www.oldwayspt.org/programs/mediterranean-program, www.eatingwell.com

- **What is it?** The Mediterranean diet comes from the traditional eating patterns of Crete, Greece and southern Italy. The common features include high intakes of vegetables and fruits, pulses (beans), whole grains, nuts and seeds, olive oil as the main fat source, and low intakes of processed/red meats and sugars. This is a whole lifestyle approach and also emphasises the importance of rest, physical activity and enjoying food and meals with others.

- **Does it work?** Research suggests this is a very effective approach for lowering risks of cancer and heart disease and living a longer life. Although this eating pattern tends to be higher in healthy fats it does *not* seem to increase the chance of weight gain. It is still unclear whether a Mediterranean diet that also encourages portion control is better for managing weight (i.e. food types and amounts) than one that just focuses on changing food types.

The principles of eating well

There is no single approach to changing eating that suits everyone. It's often a matter of experimenting to work out which is most likely to work for you. You might try out any of the dietary treatments above or might prefer to use your own self-styled approach.

Whatever you choose, it isn't essential to make all of the changes all of the time; you're not trying to achieve the 'perfect' way of eating. Modest changes sustained over time will improve diet quality and help manage weight.

Here are some of the important principles to consider in choosing specific food changes.

Plenty of vegetables and fruit

Fruit and vegetables are packed full of vitamins and minerals important in preventing a whole range of diseases including heart disease, cancer and diabetes. Most people don't eat enough of them and they can be helpful in managing weight. They are naturally bulky foods that help fill you up and are generally low-calorie.

Vegetables are particularly important at meal times. Filling half your plate with vegetables or salad is an important healthy habit. Increasing the portion of vegetables on your plate while decreasing the portion of meat, for example, will lower the calories, improve the nutrition quality but at the same time keep the total quantity of food the same so you don't feel you're eating any less. This is important, as cutting down too much on all food can leave you feeling physically hungry shortly after a meal and make managing weight more difficult.

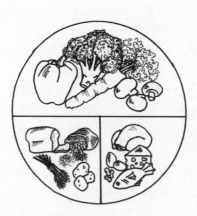

The plate above shows a healthy balance of food choices, with about half of it filled with vegetables, a quarter with starchy foods like potatoes or rice or pasta (whole grain if possible) and a quarter with lean proteins such as chicken, fish or lean meats.

If you want more details of what 'plenty' of fruit and vegetables means in practice check out the table below. To improve our health and reduce risk of various diseases at least five portions of fruit and vegetables a day is recommended. The more varied your choice of fruit and vegetables, the more likely you are to get a wide range of all the vitamins and minerals and gain more health benefits. In general, the more brightly coloured and darker the fruit and vegetable, the higher the number of the protective nutrients it contains – try a mixture of bright red, yellow, orange and dark green fruit and vegetables.

A portion of fruit or vegetables for an adult is about 80g. Here's a rough guide to one portion:

Vegetables – raw, cooked, frozen or tinned: 3 heaped tablespoons

Beans/pulses such as lentils, chickpeas: 3 heaped tablespoons (only count as 1 portion per day)

Salad: 1 dessert bowlful

Grapefruit/avocado: ½ fruit

Apple, banana, orange and other similar-sized fruit: 1 fruit

Plums and similar-sized fruit: 2 fruit

Grapes, cherries and berries: 1 cupful

Fruit salad, fresh, stewed or tinned fruit in fruit juice: 3 heaped tablespoons

Dried fruit (raisins, apricots, etc.): 1 tablespoon

Fruit juice/smoothies: 1 glass (150 ml) (can only count as a maximum of 1 portion/day)

Remember that:

- Potatoes/yams, cassava and plantain don't count as a vegetable because they're classed as a starchy carbohydrate (with bread and other cereals).
- Fruit juice/smoothies and vegetable juices count as a maximum of one portion a day.
- Beans and pulses only count as a maximum of one portion a day, however much you eat, although these are a healthy low-calorie source of protein.

Adapted from the Food Standards Agency

If you've been keeping a record of your eating habits you'll be aware of roughly how often you eat fruit and vegetables. If you eat very few at the moment, increasing to five portions a day might be a bit unrealistic at first and difficult to sustain. You may want to set more realistic short-term targets such as eating one portion of vegetables and one portion of fruit every day and then building up gradually from there. Of course, if you are already eating five portions and want to increase further, then this is fine. In many Mediterranean countries it's common to eat about eight to nine portions of fruit and vegetables a day. However, it is wise to be careful about the amount of fruit juice and smoothies drunk in a day. Litres of these can provide quite a lot of natural sugars (calories) without the bulk and fibre that the fruit itself provides.

If you choose to increase your intake of fruit and vegetables, then you also need to be specific about exactly how you might do this. In other words, what would be the best, most enjoyable and realistic way? Below are some examples of what people have done to increase fruit and vegetables in their diet. Some of these suggestions might sound promising to you, others may not. You will probably be able to come up with some inventive ideas of your own.

EXAMPLES OF WHAT OTHERS HAVE TRIED AND FOUND HELPFUL

- Adding bananas, kiwi fruit, grapes or strawberries to breakfast cereal. Maybe try frozen fruit as it's cheaper and convenient.
- Having a salad before or with a main meal – try cherry tomatoes, sliced peppers, beans and a healthy dressing, or a carrot and raisin salad.

- Keeping a bowl of fruit on the desk at work.
- Adding extra vegetables or pulses to soups, stews and casseroles.
- Chopping fruit like bananas or berries into yoghurt or jelly.
- Adding salad vegetables to sandwiches.
- Eating vegetables like carrots, cucumber and cherry tomatoes on their own or with low-fat dips.
- Having a small packet of dried fruit as a snack.

Linda had always said she hated fruit and vegetables, thought they were a hassle to prepare and that they went off before she got around to using them. But once she had decided she wanted to work on increasing the number and range of vegetables and fruits she ate, she made a specific plan. She'd buy a bag of frozen peas, sweet corn and broccoli at the supermarket every other week, a stock of tinned vegetables for when her supplies ran low, and at least one fresh vegetable each week. Sometimes this was one of her favourites like parsnips, but at other times she would buy something new and different – purple sprouting broccoli became a favourite, as did mange tout. Whatever fresh vegetables she had bought would be used first before they went off. She made a decision to focus on two main changes: to include at least one portion of vegetables with her evening meal and to have a piece of fruit with breakfast each day. On some days it didn't quite work out, but on many days it did, and it was easier than she'd imagined. At first she thought vegetables would take ages to prepare but microwaving and steaming them proved quick and easy.

Linda's story is a good example of how keeping changes realistic and thinking through the obstacles can really help improve eating habits.

Choose whole grains

Whole grains are the healthiest types of cereal and eating enough of them is important as they are known to reduce the risk of a whole range of diseases linked with excess weight.

BUT WHAT EXACTLY ARE WHOLE GRAINS?

Whole grains are cereal foods that include all three components of the grain – the bran, the starchy endosperm and the germ. There are a wide variety of whole grains, including the cereals rye, wheat (including spelt, emmer and faro), brown, red and black rice, barley (not pearled), maize (sweet corn) and oats. There are also pseudo-cereals such as quinoa, amaranth, buckwheat and wild rice that are technically not cereals but which are used in the same way in the diet and are classified as whole grains.

What happens to these grains during processing determines whether they remain whole grains or become refined carbohydrates. Many of the protective vitamins and minerals are found in the outer part of the grain and the more refining that occurs, the fewer protective nutrients they contain. For example, whole wheat is milled to produce wholemeal flour and if further processed produces white flour. Wholemeal and whole grains are very similar in their nutritional content, while white refined flour contains fewer protective vitamins and minerals.

Eating whole-grain higher-fibre foods helps protect against a whole range of diseases including cancer and heart disease as well as helping to keep the gut healthy. These foods add bulk and may help to keep people feeling fuller for longer.

Here are a few ideas that other people have tried in order to include more whole-grain foods in their diet:

- Substitute refined with whole-grain options, e.g. white rice with brown rice and couscous with bulgar/bulgur wheat.
- Add new whole-grain foods, e.g. add barley (not pearl) or sweet corn to soups and stews.
- Choose whole-grain snacks, e.g. popcorn or wholewheat crackers
- Gradually substitute white flour with whole-meal in recipes.
- There are lots of resources on including more whole grains in the diet available at www.wholegrainscouncil.org

HOW MUCH IS 'ENOUGH'?

How much whole-grain cereal and bread to include in your diet will vary from person to person. If you want to find out more about your individual needs check out: www. bdaweightwise.com.

Some recommendations suggest at least three servings of whole grains a day is needed for the associated health benefits. For more information on what one serving looks like check out the British Heart foundation website (www.bhf. org.uk) and search for 'portion guides'.

Breakfast and snack times are often good opportunities to increase the number of whole grains eaten. You might like to try whole-grain or high-fibre breakfast cereal, porridge, whole-grain toast or muffins for breakfast, or low-fat popcorn, muesli sprinkled over yoghurt or wholemeal crispbreads or crackers for snacks. Some of these ideas may appeal while others may not. The important point is to experiment and find what works for you.

Although whole-grain foods are a healthier option than refined bread and cereals, that doesn't mean white bread, pasta and rice are unhealthy foods and should not be eaten. As with all food changes, it is a matter of trying to improve choices and not attempting to follow the perfect diet. It may be that you love white bread and couldn't enjoy wholemeal bread on a regular basis. In this case, swapping a sugar-coated breakfast cereal for porridge, bran flakes or Weetabix might be a better alternative to increase the amount of whole grains eaten.

Choose fish, pulses and lean meats

Most people don't eat enough fish, yet this is a highly nutritious food that can improve the quality of the diet and help manage weight. As well as being a rich source of protein and vitamin D, it is also an important source of healthy unsaturated fats. Eating one to two servings of un-fried fish each week has been linked with a reduced risk of heart disease and stroke. The greatest benefit comes from substituting less-healthy protein sources such as fatty and processed meats with fish or seafood.

A palm-size piece of fish is considered one serving, but for more details on serving sizes, again check out the British Heart Foundation's online 'portion guides' at: www.bhf. org.uk.

Pulses like baked beans, kidney beans, chickpeas and lentils are an excellent, cheap, low-calorie source of protein and have been shown to help in managing weight and improving heart health, but most people eat them very infrequently. For further information on how to use pulses, and recipes and preparation ideas, take a look at: www. pulse.org.

As part of weekly meal planning it can be helpful to think about including two fish-based meals each week as well as at least one that includes pulses.

Choose healthy fats

Fat plays an important role in our bodies and is not the 'demon' it is sometimes portrayed as. However, eating too much fat increases the chance of gaining weight and limiting it is usually one of the key changes to consider in managing health and weight. The type of fat chosen is also important, as replacing foods high in saturated fats (e.g. fatty meats, butter, coconut oil) with those high in unsaturated fats (e.g. oily fish, olive oil, rapeseed oil) has positive effects on heart health.

There are a number of reasons why fat seems to play a role in weight control:

- Fat doesn't fill us up very well. It is a very rich source of calories and the body seems to have a poor natural ability to control how much high-fat food we eat. We tend to eat a set amount of food each day, so if that food is high in fat we will get far more calories than if it were high in vegetables and whole grains. This is sometimes part of the explanation as to why people may be struggling to control weight and yet not eating large quantities of food – the food they are eating may be high in fat (which is not always obvious) and therefore concentrated in energy (calories).
- Fat is stored by the body very easily and efficiently, more so than protein or carbohydrates.
- Fat certainly adds taste to the food we eat, and this makes it easier to eat more of it without necessarily noticing.

> • A high-fat way of eating that includes large amounts of animal or saturated fats such as fatty meats, high-fat dairy foods, fried foods and butter is linked with increased risk of heart disease and cancer.

Swapping some high-fat foods for lower-fat alternatives may be a useful way of cutting down on fat. There are no hard and fast rules and you don't have to buy low-fat everything (although you can if this suits you) or deprive yourself of high-fat favourites. High-fat food can still be eaten as part of a healthy diet; you just need to be aware of how much is consumed.

So, it is important to be aware of which types of food contain large amounts of fat. Sometimes this is obvious, sometimes not. These are some of the high-fat food choices to think through:

> • Fatty meats – the obvious fat on the outside can be trimmed, but other meats like salami, tinned ham and sausages have fat added to them in production
> • Butter and margarine
> • Cakes and biscuits
> • Fried food
> • Mayonnaise and salad dressings

Reading food labels will also help you to really understand the amount of fat in various manufactured foods. More on this later in this chapter (page 207).

Portion sizes

As we discussed in earlier chapters, portion sizes of many manufactured foods have increased substantially over recent years. This is likely to have influenced people's struggle with weight gain.

Larger portion sizes are now common in a whole range of different snack foods, manufactured products and meals served in restaurants, to the point where large portions are becoming the norm. We know most people will finish the amount of food they are served regardless of whether it is a large, average or small portion.

Larger portions are often perceived as better value, but it is important to be aware of how this can interfere with your plans to manage weight. Look out for 'big eats', 'king size', 'X% extra free', 'buy one get one free' offers or 'eat as much as you can'. Although they seem to offer value for money, it's unlikely to be beneficial to your health unless the offer relates to fruit, vegetables or whole-grain cereals – and it invariably doesn't.

If you want more guidance on portion sizes, check out www.bdaweightwise.com and the British Heart Foundation portion guides at www.bhf.org.uk (search for 'portion guides').

Soft drinks and alcohol

Alcohol is very high in calories and can prevent weight loss. For health reasons it is suggested that men and women drink no more than fourteen units of alcohol a week and spread this out evenly over three or more days. A unit of alcohol is a small glass of wine, half a pint of beer or lager or one pub measure of spirits or sherry. For more information on alcohol units check out: www.drinkaware.co.uk.

Keeping within these health limits is often sufficient for people to also manage weight, although for some people it may be necessary to restrict alcohol further. Apart from the calories in alcohol itself, drinking tends to make people feel hungrier, leading to difficulties in coping with planned food changes.

Alcohol can readily become part of someone's way of relaxing or coping with certain uncomfortable feelings. A couple of glasses of wine at the end of a long day isn't an issue if it happens intermittently but it's easy to be unaware or lose track of how much alcohol is being drunk and for what reason. Awareness of alcohol intake is important and tracking alcohol intake for a period of time is a useful starting point. More information on how to do this and Drink Aware's track and calculate alcohol app can be found at www.drinkaware.co.uk. If alcohol is being used as a way of relaxing, reducing anxiety or altering mood then consider alternative methods of addressing these needs and if concerned discuss with your family doctor.

Of course, alcohol can be included as part of a healthy diet and it isn't necessary to stop completely unless you've been advised to do so by your doctor. However, if your alcohol intake is higher than you would like here are a few ideas that others have used to help reduce their drinking. Some of these may be helpful or you may prefer to come up with your own ideas.

- Using an alcohol tracker to check on the number of units drunk
- Limiting involvement in rounds when drinking socially so everyone can choose when they drink and how much
- Alternating alcoholic drinks with a non-alcoholic calorie-free drink
- Having a couple of alcohol-free days each week
- Choosing half-pints, small glasses of wine or single shots
- Diluting alcohol with sugar-free mixers to make drinks last longer
- At home, using an alcohol measure to check how much you are pouring

Soft drinks and mixers can be full of sugar, with some canned drinks containing 7–10 teaspoons per 330ml. If drunk in large amounts, sweetened drinks can interfere with weight loss. Research in children suggests that such drinks may play a very important role in weight gain. It's thought that our body doesn't recognise the sugar and calories from drinks in the way that it would from food. So, if sweetened soft drinks are a regular feature in your diet it may be worth considering making a change. Water, unsweetened tea and coffee and herbal teas can be drunk regularly, and diet drinks and sugar-free squashes may be helpful in reducing sugary soft drinks. The precise role of sweeteners in health and weight isn't completely clear. Although there is research suggesting they are safe, they can lower intake of added sugars and have modest effects on lowering weight, some early research suggests they may have negative effects on appetite and gut bacteria. However, a lot more research is needed to really understand their role in more detail.

Understanding food labels

Making sense of food labels isn't easy but it is a helpful skill in making truly informed choices about which products to buy.

It is certainly better than trusting the manufacturer's promises on the front of the package. Manufacturers are given guidelines about using nutritional claims on the front of their products, but it is always wise to turn the product over and check what it really contains.

These are the guidelines given for fat-related claims:

- Low-fat products should contain less than 3g of fat per 100g.

- Fat-free products should contain less than 0.15g fat per 100g.
- Reduced-fat products should contain less than three-quarters of the fat in the original product.

Take a look at the nutrition labels below taken from a packet of reduced-fat digestive biscuits and a pack of standard digestives.

At first sight they may look terribly confusing. In fact, for managing weight only some parts are important. The key is to keep things simple and to look initially only at total fat (sometimes just referred to as 'fat'), 'of which sugars' and calories. Calories on nutritional labels are referred to as 'kilocalories', 'kcal' for short.

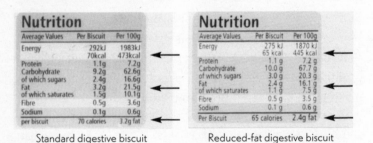

Standard digestive biscuit   Reduced-fat digestive biscuit

As a general guide, low–fat food contains less than 3g fat per 100g and high-fat food contains 20g or more per 100g. The aim is to compare products and choose the option with the lowest fat, sugar and calorie content.

The easiest way to compare these two labels is to look at the 'per 100g' column. Compare the 'total fat', 'of which sugars' and the 'calories' per 100g. The reduced-fat version has 16.1g of fat, 20.3g of sugars and 445 kcal, and the standard 21.5g fat, 16.6g of sugars and 473 kcal. This means that choosing one reduced-fat digestive (about 14g each) will only save 2g fat and 5 kcal compared to the standard biscuit – hardly the calorie-free option they are sometimes perceived to be, and they are a bit higher in sugar. This is very common in many reduced-fat sweet foods such as cakes and biscuits, where the fat content has been reduced but extra sugars or other carbohydrates have been added to ensure the taste of the lower-fat product remains comparable. So, the bottom line is that you may be eating a lower-fat biscuit, but its calorie count is very similar to the original, so it isn't really going to be helpful in managing weight.

However, there are some lower-fat foods where the differences compared to the original are greater than the above example, and such foods can be more helpful in limiting fat and calorie intake. Examples of some of these foods include lower-fat spreads and fat-free salad dressings. The choice of whether to use any of these products depends on whether you feel this would limit your enjoyment of various foods and if such changes seem sustainable. If you love a particular high-fat food and can't bear the thought of changing to a lower-fat version, then consider other ways of making healthier choices.

There is no one dietary approach for managing weight that suits everybody, with different treatments being helpful to some and not to others. Experimenting to find the approach that works for you and how to overcome the challenges that will arise in keeping new food habits in place is an essential part of this process. However, it is important to choose dietary changes that will not only help you to lose and maintain weight but will also promote foods known to be protective for health – principally more vegetables, fruit, fish, pulses and whole-grain cereals. A summary of the key points to consider in making successful long-term changes to eating is presented below.

CHAPTER SUMMARY

- Use food monitoring to increase awareness of eating and identify the triggers to eating more than planned (*see chapter 3*).
- Establish a regular eating pattern. Skipping meals often leads to difficulties with portion control or food choices later in the day. There are no rigid rules about what time to eat, although many people find their body needs food every three to four hours.
- Thinking through previous attempts at changing eating habits can be helpful in working out what was helpful and what was not.
- Food changes need to be realistic and sustainable.
- Small changes added together make a big difference over time.

- Allow time for changes to eating habits to occur. Changing any type of behaviour is complicated and requires a fair bit of experimenting.
- Avoid striving for perfection. It isn't necessary to follow the 'perfect' diet in order to manage weight. Instead, try to find a better way of eating that you are happy to continue with long-term.
- Planning ahead helps ensure healthy foods and meals are available. This avoids the need to buy food on impulse or grab whatever might be available at the last minute.
- Whatever method you choose, more fruit and vegetables, more whole grains and fewer fatty foods is the basis for all healthy approaches to managing weight.
- Portion sizes are a very important aspect of eating more healthily. Over recent years standard portion sizes have become larger, providing extra calories without people really realising this is happening.

6

Making the changes
in daily life

*I thought that this book was about changing habits. But
I've got halfway through and I haven't actually done
anything yet! I want to get on with it!*

*There are a lot more things that I need to sort out before
I can begin to change. It's all very well talking about
changing eating and activity, but I have lots of emotional
issues that need to be fixed first.*

Some people, quite rightly, want to get on with things at
this point. It is now time to do so. This chapter covers the
process of beginning to change your life.

This may seem a little too soon to some – what if there
are issues to deal with concerning emotions and other people
(*chapters 7 and 8*)? However, there are only so many things that
can be worked out in advance. There comes a time when it's
better to get started and then deal with the remaining issues
when they come up. Now is the time to begin the tricky but
exciting process of trying out new things in your life.

Making plans that will work

The key to weight management is finding plans that work for you. Not all plans will work. This is not a problem! In this chapter you will develop your abilities at being creative, making good plans and solving problems. You will start to work out what works for you.

Of course, there are plans that clearly will not work. It is worth being able to spot these, so that you can save time and avoid getting discouraged. For example, saying, 'I plan to cut down on the calories a bit' is so vague that it's probably useless. How would you know if you were succeeding or not? How much, exactly, is 'a bit'? Equally, plans can be very clear but unlikely to work. If you planned to spend two hours in the gym every night of the week (and decided that your family would just have to put up with it), you would be unlikely to keep it up for very long.

To succeed you need a plan that is sensible, clear, realistic and designed to fit into your life. Happily, everybody can come up with plans like this, as long as they follow a few simple suggestions.

Weaving the changes into your daily life

If a person wants to lose a significant amount of weight for the long term, they will have to make clear changes in their life. However, this does not mean they have to turn their life inside out. We know big plans often fail quite quickly. There is a smarter way to change habits: make changes that fit into their daily life and schedule. Instead of breaking up their usual routine, a person can look at their routine and work out how to make changes that fit into it – or even take advantage of it. Habits can become part of a regular and simple routine. Most people brush their teeth, for example, as part of their morning schedule. There are a few important points to think about here:

1. Most people do not think that brushing their teeth is a huge effort.
2. Most people do it automatically, without thinking about it.
3. People do not often forget to brush their teeth, even if their routine changes (for example, if they are on holiday) because it is a really strong habit and a part of their personal morning or evening routine.
4. When we were children, it may have seemed like a real hassle to brush our teeth. However, when it became a habit, it became no problem at all.

It would be great if eating and activity habits could be like this! Of course, eating and activity habits are a bit more complicated than tooth-brushing, but they can also fit flexibly into a person's life.

Many people find it hard to include a period of activity in their day, for example, yet, as we have seen, it may only take a small adjustment to make significant changes. For example, a person could walk more on their way to and from work. Most of us have opportunities in our week when we could walk rather than drive or be a passenger.

This is a good example of smart change from the inside out.

The principle also applies to some issues around eating. For example, if a person decides that lunch with their friends is a time when they are likely to eat too much, they can either cancel the lunches or try to arrange a change of venue to a place where there are many more healthy options on offer. One solution would break their routine, and miss out on spending time with friends, whereas the other would work within that routine. This is the approach that is helpful: to try to 'go with the grain' and where possible fit a plan into the natural course of your life.

'But I don't have a routine!'

However, some people may not be able to benefit from these ideas as much as they would like, as they do not have much of a daily routine.

This is a tricky situation, as a person is more likely to find it difficult to succeed with weight management if they do not have any routine at all. Eating needs to happen fairly regularly – if there are long gaps between meals, a person may become very hungry and this increases the risk of overeating. Equally, if a person just 'grazes' and snacks the whole time without any meals they will probably gain weight. Activity also has to happen regularly if it is going to work – not just occasionally, or lots in one week and none in the next. You can use all of the planning tools below to get you started.

It can also be that sometimes we don't like the idea of having a routine; perhaps it sounds boring or makes us want to rebel. If you feel like you tend to rebel against routine it can be helpful to recall chapter 1 on motivation where we discussed how having some sort of structure and rhythm in life can give much greater freedom in the long run. The advantage of having some sort of a routine is that it plays a huge role in building habits. Habits are formed by repeating a behaviour, most quickly if this behaviour is repeated at a similar time and place. For example, brushing your teeth in the morning in the bathroom happens at a certain time and place. You wouldn't necessarily think of brushing your teeth at other times of the day when you are in the bathroom, or at a similar time when you are in the kitchen. The repetition helps to form neural pathways in our brain and by linking a behaviour with a time and a place, the time and the place become a cue so that our brains literally have to use less effort to remember to do something. Using structure to build habits leads to greater freedom in the long run, as we spend less time thinking about doing something and having to remember to do it.

SMART planning

Sometimes, planning is fairly easy. However, when it comes to changing habits, a little more effort is required. Very often, habits around eating and activity can be quite 'stuck' because we've been doing them for so long. Also, it can be hard to know whether you have made any effective changes or not. This is why the SMART method of planning can be useful. SMART is a way to remember what makes a good plan. It stands for:

S	Simple (and specific)
M	Measurable
A	Agreed (and achievable)
R	Realistic
T	on a Timescale

If a plan is all of these, it has the best chance of success. Here is an explanation of each category.

Simple (and specific)

This means that a plan is very clear and precise, but not complicated. Vague plans generally do not work. For example, as mentioned earlier, 'I will cut down on chocolate a bit' is quite vague and it would be hard to know whether you were succeeding. However, 'I will swap chocolate for fruit and yoghurt three days a week' is a specific plan. It is also simple, which is essential. If you are going to be able to stick to it in the middle of a busy life, it's best if it isn't complicated.

Measurable

Remember Amounts Count in chapter 3 (page 104)? If a person is going to make a change to their eating or activity patterns, it is critical to be able to answer questions like 'How much?' or 'How often?' Someone might decide that they want to 'walk a lot more', but if they do not make clear how much more they are planning to do, they will probably end up doing a lot one week and much less the following week. Make sure you are clear about amounts in your planning. For activity, using an app, wearable device or pedometer/step counter can make measurement much easier, accurate and fun. In the same way, food diary apps such as Carbs and Cals or My Fitness Planner can be helpful and use food photographs to identify food portions/amounts and provide instant feedback on the nutritional content of foods.

Agreed (and achievable)

This reminds you to check that you have enough support to do your plan. Are your surroundings set up so that they will support your plan? Do you have the support of the people who might affect your plan? Can you do something about this? (More on this in the next chapter.)

Realistic

This is one of the most important parts of a good plan. It must be realistic. This means being sure that it is not too difficult or too ambitious. It's better to start small than to go for a huge project. You can then achieve your goals and move on to more ambitious things. However, if you plan big things and then fail, you have lost time that you could have spent on a good plan and probably become discouraged into the bargain.

Another recommendation is to make plans about what you *are* going to do, rather than what you are *not* going to do or have, particularly when it comes to food. For example, having a goal that you are going to stop eating biscuits at work is probably going to be more difficult to stick with than planning on swapping biscuits for fruit, not least because you might get hungry or feel deprived if you are used to having biscuits.

On a Timescale

There are two parts to this. First, when will your plan start? Second, when will you check if it is working? Successful planners always decide on exact dates for both of these events. Checking is essential – if you find you are achieving your plan easily, then you might decide to move on to something more challenging. On the other hand, if it's not going at all well then you need to try to work out what's going wrong. Checking makes sure that you will not struggle on with a bad plan for ever.

When you are thinking about when to check your plan, remember that new habits can take some time to get used to. However, it is still a good idea to check your plans after two to four weeks to make sure you are on track, and make adjustments if you are finding your goal too hard or too easy.

Write down when you are going to review your plan in your diary or on your calendar. If you don't have any kind of diary or calendar, use whatever method you would usually use to remember important appointments. Setting up electronic reminders on your phone or computer when you set your goal can be really helpful.

Some examples

Hopefully, you now have some idea of how to make SMART plans. In addition, it's very useful to see some SMART planning in action. Here are some ideas that weren't very SMART, but became SMART with a bit of thought:

A NOT-VERY-SMART PLAN

I'm just going to eat less. Of everything.

A SMART PLAN

Starting next week, I am going to cut down on portion sizes for my main meals. I will choose slightly smaller plates to put my food on and I'll fill half my plate with vegetables to add some bulk. I'll carry on having biscuits with my coffee at work, but I will limit myself to two a day and will make sure I stop working for a few minutes so I really taste and enjoy them. Nothing else changes

– I'm going to keep it simple and try not to break up my routine too much. I'll do this for four weeks and see how I am doing.

ANOTHER NOT-VERY-SMART PLAN

Walking is good, and I don't mind doing it. I'm definitely going to walk more and see how it goes.

A SMART PLAN

Walking is good, and I don't mind doing it. Starting next week, I am going to go for a 10-minute brisk walk at lunchtime, rather than just sitting at my desk and eating my lunch. I'm also going to make sure that I get one long walk in at the weekend. I don't mind when it is – I'm going to keep that flexible – but it will definitely happen, and it will last for at least 45 minutes. I'll try this for three weeks and see how it is going. I'll be interested to see whether I am a bit fitter – and enjoying it – or whether I need a bit more variety in my activity routine.

Some people may think that detailed planning is a good idea in the workplace or at home but not when changing personal habits. They may believe that these habits can be changed by sheer determination and strength of will, but in our experience planning is really important for successful habit change. It's always worth bringing some curiosity and sense of experimentation to this process to find out what works for you.

Temptations and bad ideas

There is one final point about planning to think through.

Is it more helpful to try new plans for behaviour change or stick to methods that have worked before?

It's only natural to look at what has worked before. However, it is important to be very careful when thinking about this.

Pete likes the ideas in this book but in the past he had some short-term success with extreme weight-loss methods:

> *Weight loss is incredibly difficult for me – but I do know something that works. I can lose two stone fairly fast if I follow this particular diet. It's pretty simple and easy to stick to. Thanks to reading this book, this time I'm going to focus on exercise as well. And I can use all of the stuff about thoughts and motivation to keep going. If I keep to these fairly simple (and very small) meals and steer clear of chocolate, I can keep it up. Unfortunately, the moment I go off-track – or eat even a bit of chocolate – then I tend to be in trouble. So, I'll stick to my routine. I've got to do what works best for me.*

Clearly, Pete is trying to use what he has learned in the past. Unfortunately, from the outside, it doesn't look like his favourite diet does 'work'. It might be that he has lost weight three times before by using it. Unfortunately, each time he put it all back on, plus a couple of extra pounds. Looking at it from this angle, Pete would probably realise that his diet doesn't work – it has failed, again and again, to give him weight loss for the long term.

It is important for you to have faith in your own judgement about the way you manage weight. However, it's always a good idea to be cautious about extreme weight-loss methods. They may look good and promise fast results, but so do a lot of other plans that don't work in the long term.

Don't wait – start planning now

You may already have some good plans in your head for changing your habits. However, you might need a bit more time to get ready. It's important to have faith in your own ability to plan. Remember that no one knows your life better than you do. However, if you are really stuck for ideas, don't worry, there are some tips further on in this chapter.

If you have any ideas, or beginnings of ideas, start to make them clear. It is important to write everything down. Even if your ideas are not very clear right now, try to make a start and see what happens.

- One plan for activity/exercise
- One plan for eating

You can write your plans on the planning form on page 226. This form makes you think in a SMART way and gets your ideas down on paper. There is another blank copy of this form in Appendix I, so that you can use these forms as often as you need to. You can also download them via the online version of the book, at: https://overcoming.co.uk/715/resources-to-download.

Once you've written them down, you do not need to start all four plans at once. It's up to you to decide which to start with and how many to try at any one time. However, there are a few good ideas to follow in deciding what to start with:

1. Pick a plan or plans that look the easiest and are most likely to succeed. You can always add more changes later if it's too easy.
2. Make sure you have a mixture of activity plans and plans about food. The smart move is to do both. This is what the the NWCR experts (see page 16) did.
3. Don't wait. There are always lots of (unhelpful) reasons to start 'some other time'. If your own reasons (from chapter 1) tell you that managing weight is worth doing, then it's worth starting right now.

There has been lots of research into how digital technology, and specifically smartphone apps, can help change behaviour. We would recommend considering using apps to support your goals and have included some further information about this in Appendix I.

What to do if you are dreading getting started with your plans

If the thought of starting your plans is really frightening or you find that you are making lots of excuses not to get started, check through the following:

THOUGHTS

Catch your thoughts and keep catching them. Keep a particular lookout for thoughts like 'This will never work' or 'This will be awful', 'I've got to do it perfectly all the time' or 'It's too much effort'. Question and expand these. Also check you have made plans that don't feel like a punishment or are too ambitious. It can be helpful to look at your plan and ask if you would suggest this to a good friend who was a bit uncertain about making changes. If not, and it seems too hard or unpleasant, it might be time to rewrite your plan to make it a little kinder.

MOTIVATION AND REASONS

Do you have good reasons to do your plan? Even more importantly, do you have your reasons in your mind whilst you are starting? If you can't remember why you are making all this effort, you will probably never get started. It might be helpful to check back through your notes from chapter 1.

ACTIVITY/EXERCISE PLANS

- What exactly is the plan? (Amounts Count!)

- What help do you need for your plan? Whose support would be helpful?

- When are you going to start, and when are you going to check and review your plan?

EATING/FOOD PLANS

- What exactly is the plan? (Amounts Count!)

- What help do you need for your plan? Whose support would be helpful?

- When are you going to start, and when are you going to check and review your plan?

REASONS

What are the good reasons for spending time and effort making these plans work?

THE WAY YOU ARE DOING IT

One reason why you might be dreading getting started is that your plan is too extreme. It might just be too hard, or too boring, or never leave room for treats. Remember, your plan should be something that you could imagine doing for the long term.

Doing it – putting the plan into practice

> *This has given me a lot to think about. I need to practise my planning skills. It's really important for me to get my plans perfect before I start – I don't want to do something that is too difficult, or not clear enough. I will keep working on my planning skills.*

> *This has given me some good ideas. The SMART ideas have allowed me to make my plan better. It's not perfect, but it is time to get on and do it anyway. There will probably be problems, but I can't tell what they will be until I try.*

Which of these two people will succeed in making serious changes to their habits over the next six months?

Once you have one or two plans that you are happy to start with, it's best to just get on with them. No one can really say how a plan will work out before it is actually tried. Therefore it's best to get on and try it. It may be much easier than you expected!

Whilst carrying out your plan, here are some good ideas to bear in mind:

- Remember your reasons. These will give you strength to keep going.
- Keep noticing your thinking patterns. Biased and unhelpful thoughts may cause you problems – spot them and then use your skills from chapter 2 to resolve them.
- Write down things that might be useful for the future – either useful things or blocks. It will help when you review your plan.
- Don't change your plan as you go along. Keep going and try to make it work. Of course, if you break your leg you may have to change your exercise plan. Otherwise, keep going, even if it's going badly, and try to write down what the problems are.
- Notice how things change over time. Are the changes getting easier? Is anything about your appetite or fitness changing?
- If you have a smartphone, consider using a 'habit' app; it can help you by giving you 'prompts' to stay on track. See Appendix I for more.

These are pretty much the only things to keep in mind whilst doing a plan. Otherwise it's time to just get started!

Checking – how did it all go?

After a while, it will be time to check your plan. Did it go well? What could be done better? How could you solve the problems you came across?

Kirsty is checking over her two plans and is having some very useful thoughts about them:

Today is the day – it has been four weeks. I think that things have gone pretty well. I had two main plans – first, to walk further on the way to and from work, and also to have a long walk at the weekend. Second, I was going to cut down slightly on portion sizes for main meals – and put a limit on biscuits!

I think that I have done well. I have stuck to both plans about 90 per cent. It has not been perfect – bad weather stopped me from walking once or twice, and I'm really bad at controlling my portions when I'm out with friends. Anyway, apart from that it was a success and I should be proud of myself. I'm planning to take myself shopping to celebrate this weekend.

I think that it worked well to have realistic plans that didn't take up too much of my time or mess up my life too much.

There are two main things that I need to do differently. First of all, I need to work out what to do about bad weather when I'm walking. To be honest, this is not really that difficult. When I look at my reasons, they are really important — I'm not going to let a bit of rain come between me and my goals. I'll just get the right clothes and get on with it. However, the problem with eating sensible amounts when I'm with friends is a difficult one. I'm not sure what to do about this and I need to give it some more thought.

As well as having a really honest look at how well her plans went, Kirsty is thinking about what she can learn from the whole process. You can do it, too, by following the steps below.

Did you stick to your plan?

Ask yourself how well your plan went. It should have been Measurable, so it should be easy to see how successful you were. At this point the only question is whether you actually managed to do the plan — that is, whether you managed to change your behaviour. There are two things that it's *not* about right now:

IT'S NOT ABOUT WHETHER YOU LOST WEIGHT

At this point, only think about the behaviour, not about the weight. Whether you actually carried out your plan is far more important. Changing your behaviour is what is needed to control your weight in the long term, so focus on that. Remember, there may be quite a few steps to go through before you really start losing weight. Your goals might be quite small at the moment, but you can build up to bigger things later.

IT'S NOT ABOUT WHETHER IT WAS FUN DOING THE PLAN

You are doing this so that you can manage your weight, and this is really important to you. It might be enjoyable, it might be difficult – the main point is whether you managed to do it at all.

Obviously, it does matter if you struggled through your plan and it was absolutely awful and didn't get any better with time. This is unlikely to be a good plan for the long term. Otherwise, weight loss is about doing things that really matter, for seriously important personal reasons. The reasons are exactly the same whether the process is easy and enjoyable or difficult. Imagine a person who said, 'I'd love to have children – but only so long as it was enjoyable.' Or another person who said, 'I am going to register for a degree course at university – but I will only keep doing it so long as it is enjoyable.' With any important task that involves serious changes to your life, there will be good times and bad times. It is important not to get discouraged about your weight-loss plans when you are having a bad time. It could all look completely different next week.

Recognise your achievement!

If you managed to succeed with a plan, then you have done something that is worth celebrating! It doesn't matter whether it was a big plan or a small plan. If you made a good plan and then followed it, you have done well. Long-term eating and activity habits are hard to change, so recognise your achievement by treating yourself. Take yourself shopping or to see a movie – it doesn't have to be huge reward, but give yourself a treat. However, it is probably not wise to get into the habit of rewarding yourself with food, even 'healthy' food!

If you are uncomfortable with the idea of treating yourself, try to spot the thoughts that come up when you think about it. It may be worth questioning and expanding these. In the meantime, try to give yourself a pat on the back. You have done something that you didn't have to do and that will move you towards your important reasons for change. What would you say to a good friend who had managed to stick to their goal?

Think about what you can learn

Very often, plans do not go quite as you expect. Sometimes they go wrong; sometimes they turn out better than expected. Either way, there are useful lessons to be learned.

There is a simple but useful way to learn from your experiences:

> - Think about your plan and look at any notes that you made whilst you were doing it.
> - Then think about two things: what Worked Well (the WWs) and what you would Do Differently (the DDs).

The WWs are really useful. It is always a good idea to look at success – and there may be a way to weave these WWs into your next plan. On the other hand, the DDs need some more thought. You might have some ideas about what you could Do Differently, or you might be really stuck. Sometimes something just went wrong, and it is not easy to see how it could be fixed. Don't give up on these issues – we will look at them more closely later.

Decide what you are going to do next

Once you have tried your plan and analysed how it worked, you can think about what you are going to do next. This is really up to you. If you found your plan difficult, you might just want to do it again for a while. You will probably have some good ideas about how to do it a little better a second time round. Remember that the aim here is to get new habits that will last for the long term, so it's not a bad idea to keep doing the same thing until it's really easy and natural. On the other hand, it's important to move along and develop. Amounts Count – if you are going to manage your weight, then your habits may have to change quite a bit, and this will take time. Use your judgement, and remember that if things don't go well it is not a disaster, but something to learn from.

However, if something is really stopping you from carrying out your plans, it's time to use some serious problem-solving skills.

Problem-solving: the master class

Very often, you will be able to look at a problem and easily think of a solution. However, sometimes it will be more difficult. If you are going to become an expert at weight management, you will need to develop your skills at solving difficult problems. There are some simple, structured ways of thinking about problems that give a great chance of thinking up solutions.

Of course, problem-solving is not just about fixing things that have gone badly wrong. It is more about being flexible and creative. Flexibility really matters. No one will ever find a plan that will work perfectly for them for the rest of their lives. Different situations will need slightly different plans.

Research shows that regular problem-solving keeps weight off

It seems obvious that people who are flexible and can solve problems will do better at managing their weight and health. However, there is also research that shows problem-solving is particularly important for keeping weight off in the long term. People who had lost weight using CBT either attended a 'problem-solving group' that used clear techniques to solve their weight-management difficulties or they received no follow-up. After eighteen months *five times as many* of the problem-solving group had managed to maintain more than 10 per cent weight loss compared to the group without follow-up.

This is great research, but most people do not have a local weight-management problem-solving group. However, although it might be impossible to do exactly what the research group did, there is one thing that anyone can do: learn the problem-solving techniques used by the successful group and use them regularly.

Techniques for problem-solving

Trying to find a way to solve a problem is like trying to find buried treasure in a field. Imagine that you do not know exactly where the treasure is, but you are pretty sure it is there. How would you go about finding it?

1. You need to look. The treasure – or the solution to your problem – cannot be seen straight away. It will not come to you – you have to go and find it.
2. You need to be systematic. If you just started digging randomly in the field, you would not get very far. You need a clear step-by-step plan of action.
3. Don't stop too soon. With buried treasure, you might be digging just a couple of yards away from it, but you would not know that you had been close until you finally found it. It's the same with solutions to difficult problems. You might not think that a solution is possible – that is, until the moment when you see the answer.

With good techniques, you can make sure that your search

for solutions is really effective. Good problem-solving techniques only take a few steps – five, in fact.

The five steps of problem-solving

The whole process of problem–solving is easy to understand. Here are the five steps:

1. Define your problem.
2. Make up lots of alternative solutions.
3. Analyse your alternatives.
4. Try out your solution(s).
5. See how it went – and do it again! Let's take them one at a time.

DEFINE YOUR PROBLEM

In order to solve your problem, you need to be very clear about what the problem actually is. First, it needs to be something that can be solved – something fairly clear and of a fairly manageable size. If you find that your problem is really big or really fuzzy, try to break it down into smaller parts.

When you have your clearly defined problem, then ask yourself, 'Is this *really* the problem?' This may sound odd. However, let's look at it in practice. Here is **Kirsty's** problem:

> *I really don't know what to do about eating when I am out with friends. I always try to stick to my plan – which*

is to eat smaller portions. But it never happens! I see my friends quite a lot, so eating big meals when I am out with them is really beginning to add up. I don't want to stop seeing my friends. But I don't know what to do about the portions. I know what I want to do, but it just isn't happening.

Is this really Kirsty's problem? Or:

- Is it really the size of her meals or is it the type of food – if she had a huge salad, would it matter?
- Is it really the meals that she has with her friends? If she ate less for the rest of the day before she saw her friends, would a big meal in the evening matter?
- If she did more activity on that day, would the big meal matter?

You can see that if a problem is approached from a few different angles, it may look completely different.

MAKE UP LOTS OF ALTERNATIVE SOLUTIONS

Even when you have stated your problem clearly, it's hard to just 'be creative' about solutions. However, there are techniques that give us the best chance of coming up with new ideas.

One of the most important techniques is in two different stages. The first stage is where you make up alternatives. In this stage, you are just thinking up ideas. You should not be thinking about whether they will work or whether they are sensible – that comes in the next stage. For now, you just need ideas – and lots of them.

Get a piece of paper and start writing down ideas. Anything goes. No idea is too silly or too unrealistic. If you are stuck, then it is a good idea to start off with some really silly ideas. Choose something really silly and funny. For some reason, this seems to help to 'unblock' our thinking and get us moving. When you are moving, just keep going until you have *at least five new ideas* – but it would be even better if you could get ten or fifteen.

We can follow Kirsty through this process:

- Ugh, I'm really stuck with this one. OK, I will start with something silly to get myself going: I could hire a private detective to follow me and stop me if I ordered something too big!
- Wouldn't it be great if there were restaurants that only served small portions. . .?
- I could decide in advance what I was going to eat – we usually go to the same places. That way I could avoid having to make a decision 'on the spot'.
- I could eat less, or exercise more, on the day I'm going to go out. I could see it as 'paying' for my

- evening meal – I 'pay' for the meal with a good long gym session.
- I could get my friends to check whether I am eating a sensible-sized meal.
- I could get the big meal and then leave some.
- I could choose a smaller meal and promise myself I could have more if I felt like it.
- I could choose a big portion of something without much energy in it – maybe salad or vegetables.
- I could have a filling snack before I go out, so that I feel less like eating lots.
- I could eat half and ask the restaurant to wrap the remainder, so I can have it for lunch the next day.
- How about a reward – if I manage to choose sensible portions for a whole month, I will take myself shopping.
- Or maybe a punishment – if I don't do it I will give a donation to a political party that I really hate!

That's a pretty good session. There are twelve separate ideas there. Some are silly – like the private detective! – and others are not very smart, like trying to motivate yourself through punishment. But this doesn't matter. At this stage, anything goes. The process of analysing ideas comes next.

ANALYSE YOUR ALTERNATIVES

Now you have your list of ideas, it's time to make some decisions about them. There are three steps here:

1. Throw out the options that really will not work.
2. Work out how good the other options would be in the short, medium and long term.
3. Always remember that you are trying to build positive habits that will stay with you.

First, you can throw out the obviously unworkable ideas. However, you must be careful. Some ideas might seem silly but contain something positive. For example, Kirsty thought the 'small-portions restaurant' was a silly idea, but there is some reality in it.

Second, look at the other options and work out how they would actually fit into your life. Remember to think about the long term as well as the short term. Kirsty's idea of having a snack before going out seems reasonable, but how would it work in the long term? Is this a habit she wants to build into her life? There are no simple answers to this question, but it is important to think hard about your own life and habits to see what is likely to work. Remember, you are trying to build positive new habits.

Kirsty's decision-making went like this:

> *Well, I can throw out a few ideas straight away. The private detective, obviously! Also, I really don't think that I can rely on my friends to help me out with*

portion size. Most of them have their own issues with weight—

I'm not sure they could help. Also, I can't really imagine getting into the habit of leaving food on my plate. Maybe it would be a good habit, but I love food and I believe in eating what I have paid for! Also, the 'filling snack' before I go out sounds good, but knowing me and my habits, that could turn into a very bad habit fast. Taking half the meal away for the next day might work but I might feel a bit embarrassed asking.

The 'punishment' idea would work for a while, but it's not a habit that I want to build into my life. I think that there are three things I could do that would work and would become good habits. I'm going to try:

1. *Getting some exercise on days when I know I'm going out in the evening.*

2. *Deciding in advance what I am going to eat.*

3. *For the next couple of months, rewarding myself if I get it right.*

I like these options – it seems like a good habit to get more active and remember that food is not a 'problem' – it's the balance of food and activity that matters. Also, I like the habit of deciding in advance – it means that nothing really changes about my routine with my friends, I just get a little more planning and control into my food choices. Finally, rewarding myself keeps everything positive.

Kirsty has done some great problem-solving. Her ideas are sensible and would work in the long term. Of course, this does not mean that they are guaranteed to work. Ideas have to be tested in real life.

TRY OUT YOUR SOLUTION

This is the fun part. Now you get to try out a new way of doing things. The results will not always be perfect, but they will usually be different, and in a stuck situation anything new can be useful.

When you try out your new solution(s), try to make it as SMART as possible. Keep it simple and clear. Also, give it some time to work. Not all solutions – even good ones – will work overnight. However, make sure that you do get on and try it. Without actually testing it out, you will never know if it works.

SEE HOW IT WENT – AND DO IT AGAIN!

So, did it work? Could you actually make your solution happen? A perfect solution is not much help if you can't actually put it into practice. Second, did it fix your problem? If so, how well did it work? Is the problem completely solved? Or did the solution make absolutely no difference? Of course, these are not the only options. Very often, an idea will work to a certain degree, but not as well as you hoped.

If the solution *was* perfect then the problem-solving process is over for now, because the problem is solved. However, if things went badly – or just not very well – you can start the whole process again.

Don't give up if it didn't work. Imagine if any of the great scientists had given up when they had failed to solve a problem the first time. What would you think of a police detective who had just one idea to solve a criminal case and then gave up when it was clear that this idea was wrong? Remember that a solution may be very close, but you just can't see it. Also, even if you got a solution that was OK but not great, there may be an even better one close by.

But what about weight loss?

Hold on – isn't something missing? I thought this was all about managing weight!

This whole book is about managing weight. Yet we have been focusing on plans and changes in behaviour – why?

In most dieting approaches, checking weight regularly is extremely important. It is the way to check whether you are succeeding. This is not a bad idea. It forces you to face reality. However, focusing on weight leads to problems:

1. It makes people choose fast weight-loss methods.
2. If they are losing weight, they think their diet is 'working'.
3. If they are not losing weight, they think they have 'failed'.

All of these can be a problem. Losing weight, however quickly, does not mean that a diet is 'working' for the long term. Also, if a person thinks that they have 'failed' when they do not lose weight, it's easy to imagine all of the destructive thoughts that go with this.

That's why this book focuses not on weight but on changing eating and activity habits. These are what must change if weight is going to stay off for the long term. If you take in less energy in food and burn off more in activity, then weight loss *will* follow.

However, what if you are trying out your plans and weight loss is not happening? If you think that you have changed your eating and activity a lot, but are not losing weight, you will need to think about what you are doing.

In general, if plans are happening but weight is not changing, three things can be occurring:

1. You are not clear about the amount of change that is actually needed for weight loss. For example, if you a) eat six fewer biscuits in a week, b) go for a gentle 15-minute swim twice per week and c) expect to lose lots of weight, then you will be disappointed. These changes are a great start, but Amounts Count and more than this will be needed over the longer term.

2. You are not sticking to your plans as well as you think you are. Remember, we are not very good at remembering details. You may be eating more and exercising less than you think.

3. You may have missed something important about food or activity. For example, people have been

encouraged to use lots of olive oil because it is healthy. Of course, compared to some other oils, it is healthier. However, it's still fat, and if you use lots of it, you are likely to gain weight. Misunderstandings like this are very common, even in people who see themselves as 'experts' at dieting. Bear in mind that there are gaps in everybody's knowledge, including your own.

If your plans seem to be sensible but are not producing weight loss, then there are a couple of simple steps to take. First, it is useful to start recording activity and eating again. This will make it clear if your plans are being followed and if there are any confusions about amounts of food or activity. Second, it is a good idea to get some help from a registered dietitian. The problem with misunderstandings about food is we don't know what we don't know! If you do go to speak with someone about your weight, it is really helpful to take your food and activity diaries along to give them a clearer picture of what you are doing.

Also, thinking about change or trying to find out why you've gained weight might be an important part of the process you need to go through before starting to make changes, but this does not change anything on its own.

Success will need more than one change – this is a process of trying out new things, keeping up what works and changing what does not work. Problems will come up that need to be solved. Unhelpful thoughts will certainly be around, and it is a good idea to have your reasons for change clearly in your mind. This is about doing something new in a flexible way and making plans that are designed to fit well into your life. Not everything will work straight away, but that is probably not a surprise! The important thing is to try something new and to be honest about what works. With each new plan, you will become more of an expert on your own habit change.

CHAPTER SUMMARY

- Get started – sometimes it is best to just get going.
- Make SMART plans that fit into your life.
- Watch out for extreme dieting habits.
- Carry out your plan and check whether it works.
- Actively try to solve any problems that come up.

7

Eating to manage emotions

I really want to make changes and have made some clear plans, but whenever I'm bored or stressed, I just want to eat and can't seem to stop. My plans go out of the window. I feel so disappointed and don't know what to do.

You may have SMART plans about eating but what happens if your plans are knocked off course by strong emotions or cravings? This chapter helps you spot the emotions or sensations that are getting in your way – and figure out what to do about them.

Most people understand 'comfort eating', or 'emotional eating', because most of us have at some time felt low, or bored, and eaten in response to this. Sometimes people have a craving for a particular food, and only eating that food seems to stop the craving, whilst others just have a strong urge to eat and are less concerned by the type of food.

It's not surprising we eat for emotional reasons as food and eating have close ties with our feelings. From the day we are born, we are fed not only to relieve hunger but also for comfort. If a baby cries, one of our first responses is to check if he or she is hungry, and feeding often soothes. As we are growing up, many of us will have experienced food being used as a reward or a punishment: 'If you do your homework you can have some sweets.' We might have also experienced a tendency to value some foods more than others: 'If you don't eat your broccoli you can't have any dessert.' These sorts of conversations about food are not very helpful but are quite common, and many people will have been on the receiving end of them. Food also plays a key role in celebrating special occasions such as birthdays or particular holidays and can be a deeply pleasurable way for us to come together and connect. You can probably think of lots of other ways food and emotion are linked in your life. Food has much more meaning than simply being fuel for our bodies.

So, eating for emotional reasons is common and part of 'normal' eating. It only becomes a problem when food is *regularly* used to manage emotions: when emotions feel like they are driving our eating, and we find that food is the only, or the main way, we cope with how we feel. How much people overeat emotionally, how often, and how severe this is, varies a lot from person to person. If you are regularly overeating large amounts in response to your emotions, if this feels out of control, and has happened for more than a couple of months, it will probably be helpful to do some work on this.

If this description doesn't sound like it applies to you, please feel free to skip this chapter.

If after reading this chapter, you think you might need more help with emotional overeating, there is another book in this series, *Overcoming Bulimia Nervosa and Binge-Eating*, that gives more detailed advice. You might also seek support through the resources listed at the end of this book or speak with your doctor who may be able to guide you to local help. Likewise, if you think your emotions are a sign you might be experiencing anxiety, depression or another mental-health problem, it is important to get some support for this before focusing on weight management. It's common to think mental health will improve after weight loss, and to place all the focus on weight change, but it's often more helpful to treat mental health first. Not only does this improve how someone feels, it also puts them in a better position to make changes to eating and activity. Changing habits is hard work and if mood is low there's little energy available to make changes work. For mental-health support we would suggest talking to your GP or family doctor in the first instance.

Different emotions and sensations

Emotions drive how we behave in all sorts of ways, including our eating. It is important not to demonise our emotions or become frightened of how they affect us, as they serve a number of very important purposes. We often don't notice our emotions – they rumble on in the background of our lives like the weather, and we might not really pay much attention to them unless they are extreme/strong – very stormy or hot and sunny. But to begin to understand more about if, and how, your emotions are guiding your eating, it's helpful to keep in mind why we have emotions, and how to spot them.

Emotions are an important part of our survival instinct, guiding our behaviours. They happen very fast and are outside of our conscious control. They tell us what we might need in a situation, help us prepare to respond physically, and show in our facial expressions and posture so others know how to respond to us. For example, if we are in a dangerous situation, we might experience the emotion fear and certain bodily feelings such as increased breathing and tension in our muscles. The fear makes us alert and focused, and the changes in our bodies (including certain hormones being released) will give us the energy to run away or fight to keep ourselves safe. We can also respond very differently to the same situations and emotions. For example, if you have an important interview or presentation to give, feeling nervous in advance can help you concentrate, so you prepare well. Or you might feel so stressed and overwhelmed you put off doing any preparation and experience unpleasant physical sensations such as feeling sick or tense. Some people may also find this type of situation leads to overeating, perhaps as a way of putting off doing preparation, and to cope with the anxiety. It's how we recognise and respond to our emotions that can make all the difference.

Recognising emotions

To notice a link between eating and emotions, and try to do something about it, we first need to be aware of what we are feeling, and what emotions might be driving eating. There is some discussion amongst psychologists about the range and number of emotions humans can feel. The list below is a good starting point, but you might be able to think of other emotions too.

Anger	Pain	Shame
Disgust	Relief	Contempt
Fear	Sympathy	Contentment
Happiness	Boredom	Desire
Sadness	Confusion	Stress
Surprise	Interest	
Amusement	Pride	
Awe	Embarrassment	

It also seems that some emotions can blend together to form another emotion, for example anger and disgust might combine to form contempt. Which of these emotions do you tend to feel more regularly? And do you tend to find you eat when you feel them? If so, please make a note of these.

Sensations in the body

Because one of the purposes of emotions is to make us take action, or to send us a signal, they are often felt in the body. Knowing an emotion and recognising the bodily feel of it can help us recognise and respond more quickly and effectively. Below is a list of physical sensations that can be specifically linked to eating. For example, you might notice a fidgety feeling in your stomach when you feel worried. Again, circle or make a note of any that could be familiar prompts to you starting eating and add any others not on the list.

Hunger	Enjoyable tastes
Feeling sick or dizzy	Aches
Warm and comfortable	Empty stomach
Craving sensation in the mouth	Fidgety
Tiredness	Feeling full
Pain or soreness	

People often assume emotional overeating is always linked to negative emotions such as feeling sad or angry, but positive emotions like joy, excitement and happiness can also be a trigger, so make a note of these too.

Getting specific, really specific

Making a note of your emotions and the feelings that may lead to overeating is a helpful first step. To take positive action we need go a step further and get a detailed rather than vague understanding. For example, saying, 'I eat when I'm stressed' or 'I comfort eat' doesn't really pinpoint where changes can be made. **Jackie** was confident she knew what her problem was:

The main cause of my weight problem is comfort eating. After Craig was born I was miserable for a while. I ended up being stuck in the house and I tended to eat to make myself feel better. Well, that habit has stuck with me ever since and I have been overweight. There is no doubt in my mind that comfort eating is the cause of my weight problems.

Jackie might well be right but if we asked her how she could change what was happening she probably wouldn't know where to start. Certainly, after Craig's birth she had gained weight, felt miserable about this, and comfort ate. However, if we asked a few questions about what else had changed after Craig's birth we might also discover:

- She had stopped work.
- She stopped being so active at work (she had previously been a nurse, on her feet all day).
- She stopped walking to and from work.
- She stopped eating lunch in the staff canteen.
- She started eating from the cupboards in her house.
- She started snacking on food that was in her house.
- Her sleep pattern – and due to this, her eating pattern – changed.

Looking at Jackie's situation in this depth gives a much clearer idea of a whole range of things she might be able to do differently that would help address her comfort eating: having more contact with people, walking more, eating only when sat down, making sure she has easy-to-prepare healthy food in the house, meal and snack planning, and getting more support to help her sleep better could all help. We can see that Jackie's comfort eating is part of a whole host of other circumstances, circumstances that she might be able to change alongside her comfort eating.

Jackie's situation also shows it is not only comfort eating that's causing difficulties in managing her weight. Reflecting on this point, noticing what other factors might be involved and making a judgement about how much of a difference emotional overeating is really having on your own weight management is really important.

Another essential point to bear in mind is exactly what happens when you overeat. Suppose you spotted that feeling sad tends to result in overeating. What would that mean exactly? Would you just eat an extra big plate of pasta once in a while? Or would you end up snacking on big bags of crisps and sweets every evening for a couple of weeks? The extra pasta once in a while might not really be much of a big deal. However, lots of crisps and sweets on a regular basis would probably be important. Remember, Amounts Count.

Finally, was there ever a time when you were overweight but did not really have these feelings very often? And was there ever a time when you had these feelings but were not overweight? It is important to think hard about this, because if you put your effort into trying to change something that isn't that important, you could waste time and it might not affect your weight loss. Don't worry if this all sounds like quite a lot to think through, we will come back to this later in the chapter and think through some practical solutions.

How to start working with emotions and eating

When it comes to emotions, knowing what we are feeling is an important step in managing them, and you might find the more you think about your emotions and eating, the more specific links you can make between the two. If you do make connections, note these down as you carry on reading. As well as emotions, physical hunger and sleep can play a major role in unplanned overeating.

Physical hunger

Somewhat surprisingly, eating at irregular times and going for long periods without eating can be a big part of the problem. We might think it's our emotions driving us, but actually it might be something else, as **Pauline** began to realise:

> I had been trying to lose weight for quite some time and had got into the habit of skipping breakfast. I'd just have a small lunch at around 2pm or later and dinner at 8pm as a

way of not eating too much. To be honest I didn't usually feel hungry in the mornings and in the afternoons I'm so busy at work I don't really have time to think about food. But by the evening I am starving! So, I tend to pick at biscuits and bits of cheese, and whatever I'm cooking when making dinner and then I would have quite large helpings at dinner. I usually feel a bit bad about this and, because I'm trying to lose weight, will skip dessert with the family. The problem is I like to snack late into the evening – crisps, ice cream, any leftovers in the fridge. Then of course I feel bad about this and really full when I go to bed, so I make all these plans to be good the next day.

What do you think is going on here? Although Pauline wants to manage her weight, one of the main challenges she is facing is the long gaps between eating. By the evening she is physically very hungry, and her body needs food. Eating in response to hunger is one of the basic drives that keeps us alive and reminds us to eat. If someone goes for a long period of time without eating there will come a point where the thoughts of food will become very intrusive and will take over. It's a bit like holding your breath – there will come a point when you will just eat, and the choices you make at this time are less likely to be the healthy choices you had planned. This drive to eat when hungry is a normal survival instinct that can be seen in all animals, but unlike other animals, we as humans are likely to feel all sorts of emotions if we overeat, such as shame and guilt, and then try to overcompensate.

Eating regularly can be very helpful and is the first step in dealing with emotional overeating, particularly for people who are leaving long gaps between meals.

The easiest way to spot if you are leaving too long between eating is to use the Eating Record Form included in this book (chapter 3 and Appendix I). Keep your Eating Record as usual but write down the times when you are eating. It's important to try to include everything you eat, including the times when you overeat – even if this feels really difficult to do because you are ashamed or feel guilty. Keep your diary for a few days or a week and then look back over it and work out the number of hours between eating.

Do you notice any long gaps that you could link to over-eating later on? For most people, eating every 3–4 hours when awake keeps physical hunger at bay, so this could be breakfast, lunch and evening meal with a healthy snack in between, or any combination that works for you. At first that might seem like a lot of food, but the snacks don't have to be particularly large, a piece of fruit or a yoghurt is fine. Without being in some sort of regular eating pattern it is going to be very difficult, if not impossible, to stop episodes of unplanned overeating in the future.

Getting into a regular eating pattern can take some time, particularly if you are used to leaving long gaps between meals. However, if you find you are emotionally overeating, we would suggest this as the first step you need to take. Once you have got used to this you can start to work on other areas.

You might find you get a little hungry between eating, but this is fine, physical hunger is a normal sensation – it doesn't need to be prevented or avoided, just responded to, preferably by regular eating and planning.

We can also have other types of emotional hunger that can feel like physical hunger, and this is often where emotions and overeating meet. To work with emotions and overeating we need to make sure that the likelihood of being very physically hungry is reduced.

Sleep

Another physical trigger for overeating can be tiredness or lack of energy due to inadequate sleep time, or poor-quality sleep. This can increase urges to eat as we crave extra energy to keep going, and for comfort as a way of dealing with feeling sleep-deprived. Lack of sleep can also cloud our judgement, so we are less likely to make healthy choices. Finally, many people who are sleep-deprived will be up during the night, often into the early morning. The types of food chosen late at night, often sweet or high-fat foods, are usually different to those we would choose for breakfast at 8am after a restful sleep!

Lack of sleep also causes physical changes in the body, including upsetting hormonal balances such as cortisol and hunger hormones, as well as insulin sensitivity.

Of course, how to get good-quality sleep is a whole topic in itself, and to find out more about how to improve sleep you might want to have a look at another book in this series, *Overcoming Insomnia and Sleep Problems*, and the resources in the appendices.

Eating regularly and sleeping well are vital but often overlooked physical factors that have a huge impact on our emotions and managing our eating. Managing these first can enable us to then concentrate on any remaining factors that may be driving emotional eating. For some people just improving their eating patterns and sleep may be enough to reduce emotional and unplanned eating.

Emotional aftershocks

Making these links between feelings and starting or wanting to eat is really helpful. The other thing to bear in mind is we are also likely to experience emotions during and after overeating, many of which drive our subsequent behaviours. It is important to take this into account, too, as these emotions can lead us to eat even more and/or to try unhelpful extreme weight-management plans.

Here are some examples:

- Feeling so bad about body shape that a rigid 'crash' diet is tried
- Skipping breakfast because so much had been eaten the evening before and feeling a bit sick in the morning
- Not eating for many hours because of not feeling hungry and wanting to make up for overeating the day before

- Banning sweets or chocolate from the house because the cravings are so difficult
- Going to a really energetic exercise class or very long run to make up for overeating

Do any of these sound familiar? If you notice a pattern here make a note of these too as they can keep unhelpful eating patterns going, so need to be considered and managed.

Getting more familiar with your feelings

The more you analyse and understand your feelings, the more you will be able to see how they affect your life, which puts you in a better position to manage things differently. You may have spotted a large number of emotions or sensations that get in the way of your plans. However, you won't be able to deal with them all at once. It is best to choose one or two to work on, then ask yourself:

Step 1

- What makes the feeling happen? What are the 'triggers' for this feeling?
- When or where do they happen most?
- What makes the feeling stronger? What makes it weaker? Think about all of the times that something has helped the feeling go away.

- What happens when you act on the feeling? What do you do?
- Are there times and places when you have this feeling, but it doesn't spoil your plans – that is, you don't act on it?
- Has this feeling always been present? Have there been times when it wasn't there?

Emotions and sensations often affect what we do, even if we are not aware of them.

Jotting down your responses to the questions above will give you some helpful information about your emotions. This first step will take a little while and is worth coming back to. You may already have some helpful insights about some of these from the recording covered in chapter 3 and from earlier in this chapter.

Once you have more of an idea about how feelings come and go, you will be able to consider what happens when you act on them. Then you can go on to:

Step 2

- What happens after you act on an emotion by eating? Do you really feel better after doing what you felt like doing?
- If you did feel better, for how long?
- Did you feel anything else about what you did – then or later?
- What effect did acting on your feelings have on your health – and feelings – in the long term?

Here are **Pete's** responses to some of these questions:

Well, some of it is fairly obvious. I eat more because I'm in a good mood and I love the sight of good food and big portions! It's also obvious that I enjoy the food at the time and later feel way too full. So, I feel good at the time but not so good later, and then feel guilty. To be honest, I probably spend more time feeling bad about my weight than I do enjoying the food. And the truth is that if I keep doing this in the long term, I am going to gain even more weight and my health will suffer. Now I think about it, I do realise it's not the same all of the time. With some friends and some people from work, I won't overeat, even though I see exactly the same food in front of me and I have the same feelings. So, I guess it doesn't always have to be like this.

What do your answers tell you? Although everyone is different, most people find their feelings and acting on them aren't usually that helpful when it comes to eating.

Acting on these feelings makes things worse

Most people find feelings promise a lot – for example, a sad feeling might promise eating something will make you feel better – but when they think hard about what actually happens, they find they feel worse; the opposite happens. However, it's important not to forget emotions are there for a reason and ask:

- What are your feelings telling you that you need?
- What are the more helpful alternatives?

When you are going to eat outside of what you had planned, ask yourself:

- What is it I want?
- What does my body really need?
- What am I really hungry for?

Patricia had had a really busy day at work, and not much time to eat properly.

> *When I got home from work I just stood in the middle of the kitchen and started eating whatever I could find. But then I somehow remembered to ask myself 'What is it that I really need?' and I suddenly noticed how tired I felt, that my back ached, I had all these jobs on my to-do list that I hadn't done and would have to do tomorrow. I felt worried about the next day and a bit overwhelmed. I realised what I wanted was not to feel tired and stressed like this. Then I asked myself, 'What will carrying on eating do for me?' And I thought, yes it will taste nice now and it will also distract me from my work worries but it won't make me less stressed, or less tired.*

Patricia's emotions were sending her an important message, to do something about her difficult situation at work. There are a whole list of other things that Patricia could do that would actually help with her problem – having a warm bath so her body would feel better, calling a friend to talk through her difficult day, deciding if she could say something to her boss, etc., etc. Food was a temporary relief, but it was stopping Patricia taking any positive steps, and was actually just going to make her feel worse.

You might not always find it possible to know what it is you actually need, but it's certainly worth asking the question.

Emotions and sensations come and go

Earlier in this chapter we compared emotions to the weather, and, just like the weather, emotions come and go, including the ones that are causing you problems. This often depends on what is happening around you. For example, a person might have a really strong craving for chocolate, but then the phone rings. During the conversation, the 'really strong' craving just vanishes.

Will these feelings come again in the future? Almost certainly. Will they go away again? Yes, definitely. All emotions and sensations are temporary. So, another way of working with emotions is to accept they are happening but not necessarily to act on them. The fundamental truth about emotions is they don't last, unless the situation remains exactly the same, or we continue to think and focus on the situation that triggered the feelings in the first place. Even then, if we watch them closely, emotions often change. It is important to remember, though, that if we continue to think about the trigger, the emotions will often continue. For example, if we continue to worry about a difficult conversation with a friend we will continue to experience the same difficult emotions, and indeed these feelings might even become amplified.

Look at the thoughts that go with emotions

In chapter 2, we noted that strong emotions or sensations almost always bring thoughts with them, or vice versa. We have also seen how feelings tend to promise things. For example, if Patricia noticed when she came in from work that she hadn't eaten and felt tired she might have spotted the unhelpful thought, 'I've not eaten properly all day, so I need some sugar to give me some energy – I'll eat those chocolates.'

Below are a few examples of thoughts that might go with particular emotions and sensations. They are all in some way biased, unhelpful, or present a limited view of the situation. Look at this list and imagine what would happen if you just believed them without questioning them – how would it affect your weight-management plans?

Sadness	Hunger
I need something to cheer me up. Nothing else fun is going to happen, so I may as well eat something.	I'm not full yet – I need some more. I'm hungry. I need some food. This is awful. I can't bear it.

Pleasure	Cravings
I need to allow myself some pleasures! You only live once. It's better to enjoy this than worry about dieting.	I won't be able to concentrate until I have eaten this. There's no point fighting it – it doesn't work. I'm just addicted to chocolate – it's best to accept it.
Anger	**Tiredness**
It's not fair that I should have to change my eating. People who stare at me are idiots. I will eat what I like, to show them. How can I stick to my plans when they behave like that? I might as well not bother.	I need to rest. I need a snack for energy. I feel too tired to cook, I'll order a takeaway. I deserve a treat, I'm tired.
Boredom	**Anxious**
I may as well have a snack to break up the time. Meal planning is boring – I can't be bothered. All of this new food is boring – I can't be bothered.	I can't refuse seconds, they'll think I'm rude. Having something to eat will calm me down. I'll do it after I've eaten this.

Do any of these sound familiar? What thoughts go with the feelings you noticed earlier in the chapter?

It's fairly easy to see how these thoughts and feelings will get in the way of what you want to achieve in the long term. In chapter 2 we looked at how to work with thoughts that are getting in the way:

- First, spot the thoughts that seem to go with the strongest feelings. Then write them down in a way that:
  - Explains the most important part of the thought.
  - Summarises it briefly.
- Then you can then go on to: Question the thought. Expand it.

Looking back through your notes about emotions and eating, write down the thoughts that go with those emotions. If you can question and expand upon the thoughts that go with your feelings, you will be able to reduce the power of your feelings. Remember that the main goal is to keep going with your plans and work with your feelings.

Putting this into practice

Accepting emotions

Experiencing uncomfortable emotions is a natural part of life, but there is a difference between finding these emotions unpleasant and finding them so unbearable we would do anything to avoid them. When it comes to eating, food can be used in many different ways, including as a distraction from the emotion, as a comfort, as a way of dampening down or distracting, etc.

It is worth bearing in mind that you will have accepted emotions and sensations previously without eating. There will have been times when you will have done something even though you were anxious, or not said what you felt like saying to someone because it would have hurt their feelings. Have you ever felt angry but chosen not to act on it? Have you ever faced a challenge even though you didn't feel confident? Have you ever felt really happy and not eaten? There are probably many times when you have done something when you didn't feel like it or when you haven't done something despite a strong urge! Learning to tolerate and accept but not act upon emotions that are triggering the urge to eat is vital in breaking the habit of overeating.

This is a really important point. If a person has a problem with feeling sad and this makes them overeat, it might seem a sensible way to try to get rid of the sadness. However, sadness is a normal part of human life. So are anger, fear, boredom, tiredness, loneliness, hunger and lots of other feelings. Nobody can get rid of them. Emotions and sensations are our guides but they do not need to be our dictators, and they do not always direct us to the most helpful actions. They are also temporary, and you can ride them out.

Why do you want to make changes?

In chapter 1 you spent some time deciding your reasons for managing your weight. These values are important and personal to you. They can get you through hard times and when you achieve each of your goals the emotions you feel about these successes also need to be acknowledged and celebrated. Revisiting these values and reminding yourself of your reasons can be enough to break the spell of your emotions, and to prevent you from acting upon them.

Replacements and distractions

Although resisting or ignoring emotions definitely has its place, it is also helpful to find replacements or distractions.

REPLACEMENTS

By now you probably have some clear ideas about which emotions are most likely to lead you to overeat. This means you might be able to find replacements before you are even in certain situations.

Looking at your list of trigger emotions or sensations, what else could you do for yourself when these come up and you might go off-plan? Are there alternative ways to deal with tiredness or stress, to reward yourself, to celebrate? The key to replacements is to find something that breaks your usual way of responding, is pleasurable, and/or nourishing, and that doesn't include food. There have been a few examples of replacement activities already in this chapter, and **Dave** wrote the following list:

- If I have a difficult meeting with my boss I will make sure I have time afterwards to go for a 5-minute walk round the block using a route that avoids going near any shops where I could buy food.

- I will put aside time to work on my hobbies, which keep my hands busy in the evening.
- I will ask my close friend to be a support person so I can ring them up if I've had a difficult day and have the urge to eat.
- I will get into a regular night-time routine, so I am ready to go to bed on time. Include brushing my teeth by 9pm so I'm less tempted to eat.

What replacements can you think of?

My replacements:

_____

_____

_____

DISTRACTIONS

As we saw earlier, someone might have a really strong urge to eat some chocolate and then the phone rings and they forget all about it. We can engineer distractions like this into our lives, and research shows this approach, sometimes called Surfing the Urge, can be a really helpful way of dealing with cravings.

SURFING THE URGE

For most people food cravings that aren't caused by physical hunger last about 20 minutes. If we can get through these 20 minutes we will usually successfully avoid succumbing to the urge. To get through the urge you need to find an activity that takes your mind off the craving – so sitting in your kitchen thinking, 'I mustn't think about biscuits' or looking through recipe books won't help. Here are some ideas:

- Phoning a friend
- Going for a walk or doing some other form of physical activity
- Putting on some music. Music is a surprisingly effective way of changing our emotions, so it can be useful to be aware of what tracks alter your moods. Turning up the volume and dancing/playing air guitar can also help!
- Putting on a movie or playing a computer game
- Doing something productive (as long as it's a task that isn't likely to prompt an unhelpful emotion such as boredom)
- Removing yourself from the physical environment where you want to eat, for example getting out of the kitchen

OVERCOMING WEIGHT PROBLEMS

What else could you add to this list?

My distractions:

_____

_____

_____

Surfing urges helps to build our tolerance to emotions and provides alternative, more helpful ways to respond. Both replacements and distractions can also meet the need that the emotion is highlighting.

How we speak to ourselves

How we speak to ourselves about our emotions and behaviours can have a strong effect on our behaviour. On the surface it might seem like common sense that if we overeat a large amount of unplanned food in response to feeling a strong emotion, we should tell ourselves off. We've done something 'wrong' haven't we? Don't we deserve to be disciplined? Isn't being strict with ourselves how we will get back on track? Actually, there's quite a lot of evidence that shows talking to ourselves in this way has quite the opposite effect! Being self-critical and harsh tends to make

272

us feel worse about what we have eaten, or rebellious, or both, and so tends to lead to more overeating to manage these feelings.

If we think about it this makes sense. Bring to mind someone who has helped you achieve something important in the past. Perhaps a teacher or coach at school or a helpful manager at work, or if you can't think of anyone just imagine someone. Usually these people:

- Are supportive and encouraging
- Are honest about what you need to improve upon but in a constructive, not a critical way. They give clear, practical advice about what you need to change and how to do this
- Help you to try again until you succeed

This is quite different to someone telling you that you're an idiot, you've done it wrong again, and that you always fail so why are you bothering.

Which of these approaches do you think would be most effective in helping someone make changes to their behaviour and manage their weight?

Many people are quite self-critical, and this can be very ingrained, so it can be hard to think of alternative ways of speaking to ourselves. One way of looking at this differently can be to think about how you would talk to a friend or someone you care about. If a good friend rang you up and told you they had messed up something important to them, they had tried but it hadn't worked, what would you say to them? Take a moment to write down a couple of words or phrases you might say to them.

For example, you might be warm and understanding in your tone, and you might say something along the lines of:

- 'We all make mistakes, you did the best you could.'
- 'It sounds like you tried really hard, is there anything you learned from this that would help next time?'
- 'What you are doing isn't easy, but I know it's important to you, so keep trying.'
- 'That sounds really difficult, what could you do in the next couple of hours that might make this feel a little easier? And in the longer term?'
- 'I'm so sorry it didn't work this time, but I'm here for you, so keep at it.'
- 'I'm so proud of you for trying, next time it will be easier.'

Now imagine how you would feel if you spoke to yourself in a similar way the next time something didn't go to plan. It might feel a little odd to do this at first as you might be used to giving yourself quite a hard time, but it does get easier with practice. Writing down a couple of phrases can help. Many of these suggestions draw upon the work of Dr Kristin Neff and colleagues; for more information please visit https://self-compassion.org.

Pressing pause

As mentioned earlier, emotions are very fast automatic responses outside of our control but we can learn to slow down our reactions so we don't respond on auto-pilot. Building in a pause gives us time to move out of this automatic mode so we can bring in some more conscious decision-making and use some of the techniques described in this chapter. Emotions tend to fade very quickly unless we carry on thinking about whatever situation prompted them. For example, worry is often linked to thinking about a situation that might happen in the future or remembering something that happened in the past. It is unlikely the actual trigger situation is happening as you feel that emotional urge to eat. By using pause you can bring yourself back to what is actually happening in the present and make choices on what to do next based on what is happening at that moment.

So, how to pause or take time out? Taking a few deep breaths and focusing on the feeling of breathing is a useful pausing technique. Some people may find practising meditation and mindfulness approaches helpful.

Here's a specific pausing approach that may be useful and you might like to try right now – it's called the 5-4-3-2-1 grounding technique:

5. See: Look around for five things that you can see and say their names out loud or in your head, for example computer, table, book, phone, pen.

4. Feel: Notice your body and name four sensations. Say them out loud or to yourself, for example feeling your feet warm in your socks, the chair on the back of your legs, the breath at your nostrils, your hands holding this book.

3. Listen: Notice three sounds. It could be the sound of traffic outside, birds singing, or other people nearby. Say the three things out loud or to yourself.

2. Smell: Notice two things you can smell. This could be any smells around you, or if you can't smell anything at the moment then remember two smells you like such as lemon, clean washing, etc.

1. Breathe: Finally, try to notice one complete in-and-out breath wherever you feel it most in your body (the tip of your nose, your nostrils, or your belly as it rises and falls). Try to follow the breath at this place as you breathe in, saying, 'in', and then 'out' as you breathe out.

This pausing exercise can be done anywhere and can help to slow you down enough to notice what emotion you are feeling, to help accept that it has happened but that it will also fade, and then you can decide how you can respond to it helpfully.

Holding steady

It often seems easier to give in to emotions or sensations. Sometimes it is. If you have a craving for something sweet, you may just want to eat it so you can concentrate again and get on with things. It's important to be clear that sometimes this can be a relief and is OK occasionally. The problem is that if you do this frequently, in the long term it will only make things worse because it reinforces the habit of overeating in response to emotions, making it more likely you will do it again because:

1. Using food to manage feelings gives you the idea that this is the only way you know to respond to your emotions. It means you are less likely to try other more helpful alternatives, so you feel less in control.

2. The immediate relief you feel is a strong positive feeling, and food is naturally rewarding. That is why although trying to use willpower to resist your impulse to eat may work sometimes, it is usually more helpful to use the techniques described in this chapter.

The good news is that the opposite is also true. Every time you behave differently, every time you don't overeat emotionally, you are breaking the connections between eating and emotions, and learning a different way to respond.

What to do when emotions are difficult nearly all the time

For most people, negative emotions can be painful, but they are not a problem all the time. There are good days and bad days, but there is always light at the end of the tunnel. Unfortunately, some of the time, emotions like sadness, anxiety or guilt become a serious problem on their own. When strong and painful emotions are present most of the time, they may need treatment in their own right. As mentioned earlier, if they are beginning to seriously interfere in your life, then it may be time to consider getting some outside professional help.

Getting help for emotional difficulties makes sense in the same way that consulting a doctor about a medical problem or a financial advisor about money makes sense. It makes sense to consult an expert at these times. In chapter 9 there is some information on seeking professional help, finding a good therapist and using medication.

Have a back-up plan

If you have a tendency to overeat in response to your emotions, this can take some time to change. It's possible it might happen again, even if you put all you now know into action. So, it's important to consider making a back-up plan. You might think this isn't going to be necessary but thinking this through in advance, preferably now as you finish reading this chapter, can be very helpful. Emotions happen so quickly, and are not in our conscious control, so your plan needs to be in place in advance. Using this chapter, what could you do to help yourself before you are tempted to overeat? Another way to approach this is to use the problem-solving strategy discussed in chapter 6.

Here's **Jackie's** back-up plan that she keeps with her diary:

I know that the following emotions can cause me to overeat:

Stress. Worry.

When I spot the early signs of feeling like this I will (replacement and distraction):

If I know I am going to go into a situation that makes me feel stressed I will use problem-solving to work out some options.

I will be using the 5-4-3-2-1 grounding technique.
I will have a playlist of upbeat music on my phone that I will play before and after the situation. I will try to go for a walk whilst listening to a couple of these tracks.

If I do overeat then I will:

Try to draw a line under it, recognise we are all human and this happens to lots of people. If I am unkind and very critical to myself I'll try to be gentle and get back on track.

Go back over my values and why making changes to manage my weight is important to me.

Be very careful about making extreme plans in response and get straight back to a regular eating pattern.

I will try to get back on track as quickly as possible. I will try to think about what I could learn from what just happened and how I could use this in the future.

Here's a back-up plan for you to complete:

MY BACK-UP PLAN

I know the following emotions can cause me to overeat:

_____

_____

_____

_____

When I spot the early signs of feeling like this I will:

_____

_____

_____

_____

I could use the following distractions:

_____

_____

_____

I could use the following replacements:

_____

_____

_____

_____

If I do overeat then I will:

_____

_____

_____

CHAPTER SUMMARY

- Notice how emotions and sensations affect your weight-management plans.

- Spot the most important ones, name them and get to know how they affect you.

- It's important to ensure you are getting enough sleep and eat regularly so you can concentrate on the other factors driving eating.

- Make plans in advance about how to respond to emotions, as they quickly trigger an automatic reaction.

- Consider getting help if your emotions are causing you lots of problems.

- Remember feelings do pass, like the weather, and you can ride them out without eating.

8

Dealing with other people's reactions

Things got so much easier when I moved out of the house I was sharing with friends. We all ate together and picked up each other's habits. As soon as I moved out it was so much easier to eat healthier food and choose smaller portions.

I know I need to change my habits. The trouble is, so does everyone else in the family! How am I going to manage if my husband, kids and friends all carry on making unhealthy food choices and being inactive?

In an ideal world, your plans to change habits wouldn't be influenced by other people, but we know this is often not the case and the people around us can affect our choices in positive and negative ways.

This chapter helps you deal differently with some of the challenges of other people's reactions to your habit changes.

The first step is to work out the different ways in which other people are affecting you, so you know what you need to do.

How other people can influence your plans

There are lots of different ways in which other people can influence your plans to change eating and activity habits.

Let's look first at two general areas:

1. *Other people's choices affect your choices*
   For example, your housemate may choose to fill the fridge with large amounts of tempting foods or your partner might insist there isn't enough money for gym membership. In the first example you are facing an additional choice – whether to eat more of the tempting foods than you had planned – and in the second example you have one fewer choice – going to the gym. In both examples, other people have affected what you can and can't do. This can feel like a hopeless situation and can sometimes feel like there's no way out

2. *The way other people treat you can affect your choices*
   Sometimes people around you may encourage your plans to manage your weight, or they may be negative, perhaps saying your plans will never work, or they may avoid you if they know you are making different lifestyle choices. Unfortunately, there are also many examples of discrimination against those with larger bodies and this can be experienced in various ways including hurtful comments.

Here we will look at these two areas in turn. First we will help you to analyse the ways in which other people affect you. Then we will cover the skills that will help you respond to these situations.

Other people's choices can affect your choices

Jackie is thinking about the things that would make managing her weight a little easier:

> *Well, in my ideal world, it would be like this. I would have a private gym in one room of my house. And a personal trainer, of course. I would have a fridge full of healthy food. I wouldn't buy it, because I would have my own personal dietitian to pick it all out for me. And I'd have a personal cook to keep an eye on the portion sizes. Also, if I ever wanted to go out, to an exercise class, for example, then I would have someone around who could look after Craig – childcare is important. . . If I went out of the house, I would make sure I wouldn't go near any fast-food outlets, or shops that sell snacks, or anywhere else that might be challenging. Hang on, I'm sure I can think of some more things. . .*

All of this would certainly make managing weight a great deal easier, but most people's lives are far more complex – and full of other people who can influence plans. A partner, family, friends, workmates, a boss and total strangers can all affect our plans. The people who run big food businesses, the diet industry and the local shops can certainly make a difference to the choices made.

OVERCOMING WEIGHT PROBLEMS

All of these can affect you in one of two ways – either they *change your environment* in some unhelpful way, or *you rely on them* for some things and they aren't helping. Let's look at these in turn.

Other people change your environment

Your environment – the things that are or are not around you – really matter. We know the changes to our environment over the last twenty to thirty years have led to more people finding it harder to manage their weight. None of us are immune from these influences and personal surroundings can make a big difference.

Here are some examples:

- Your partner insists on having large amounts of less-healthy food in the house that you find hard to resist.
- You feel you need to have snacks in the house for children or visitors.
- Family or friends bring round tempting food and it seems rude not to have some.
- You stay with family or friends and they serve less-healthy foods.
- Your 'treat' to your children is to take them to a fast-food outlet.
- When you go out with friends, they choose restaurants with less-healthy food or insist on ordering food to share.

- Your colleagues always have a tin of biscuits in the office.
- There are vending machines with chocolate and crisps close to your desk.
- Your desk has a computer and a phone, so you never really need to leave it apart from to go to the toilet.
- You have a job that needs you to sit at your desk most of the day.
- You go out with friends to pubs and bars that only serve less-healthy foods.
- You have to go shopping with children who beg for cakes, biscuits and sweets.
- Your family is in the house watching a movie and eating snacks when you are planning to go out and exercise.
- The fast-food outlets near your home offer no healthier options.
- Some places offer free samples of food.
- In many shops near your home, there are chocolate and crisps easily available near the checkout.

There are many ways in which other people's choices affect yours. This is just a short list.

How does your environment spoil your plans for eating and activity? Think in turn about the different environments you find yourself in. Have a look at the list below. Write down the main thing in each environment that messes up your plans.

Environment	This messes up my eating plans	This messes up my plans to be more active
Home		
Work		
Friends' houses		
Family's houses		

	Restaurants, or other eating or drinking places	Other places when you are out and about	Places on journeys that you make – for example to and from work, picking up other people

Don't worry about filling every box – this is just meant to help you think about these issues in an organised way. Later, there will be some ideas on how to overcome these difficulties. Now let's look at another way in which people can affect you.

Other people do not give you practical support

It would be a lot easier to change activity and eating habits if you could do exactly what you wanted all the time. However, most people cannot do this. You may have people who rely on you – children, for instance, or other relatives. You may also rely on other people, such as on your partner to help out with things around the house. This becomes very obvious when people who want to be more active decide to do some activity. Here are some examples:

- You need your partner to look after an elderly relative whilst you do some activity.
- You need people to cover at work whilst you take a walk at lunchtime.
- You need your partner or family to agree on money – for the gym, for example, or for clothes or equipment for activity.
- You need someone to give you a lift back from the gym in the evening when it's dark.

- You need someone to look after your kids so that you can shop without them nagging you for unhealthy food.
- You need someone else to do the shopping so there is healthy food in the house, and you don't end up having to order a takeaway.
- You need someone to do their share of the household chores so you can have the time to be active in other ways.

There are many more examples like this. Later on, we will take you through how best to manage these issues. For now, it is important to understand how they affect your choices.

First of all, think of all of the situations where other people set back your plans by not helping. Think first about your plans for activity and then about eating. Ask yourself:

- Which parts of your current plans are difficult and sometimes fail because other people will not (or cannot) help?
- Which of your plans have failed completely in the past because other people have not helped?
- Which plans have you never even tried because you have always assumed that you could never get the support you need from other people?

These are the problem areas: write them down. Second, work out:

- Who is not giving you the practical support – partner, friends, colleagues?
- What exactly do you need them to do? Try to be precise.

Again, write these things down.

These are some of the practical ways in which other people can make managing weight difficult for you. However, there are other ways in which they can affect you that are less clear but can matter just as much.

How other people treat you

People encourage you – and discourage you

You may have a friend who encourages you to go out for a long walk each weekend. You may have another friend who tries to get you to go on 'crash' diets with her. You may have a neighbour who says mean things to you in the street or a housemate who is unpleasant about your plans behind your back.

We do not need to worry about the positive influence that other people have (though don't forget to thank them once in a while!), but the negative influence can be very difficult to deal with. Some people are simply unpleasant and mean – but others may be responding negatively because they are confused by what you are doing or somehow take it personally. Weight can be a very sensitive issue for many people.

If you are making plans and taking action to manage your weight it may make others feel uncomfortable, and they may act in a way that is not helpful for you. It is important to note we are talking about the *effect other people's behaviour has on you*, not judging other people or analysing what they are trying to do.

Think about your activity and eating plans. Who has a strong effect on them? Specifically, which people lead you to break your plans? Think about the following sets of people:

- Partner
- Family
- Friends
- People at work
- Strangers
- Any others?

Write down who seems to have a big effect on you. Remember, this does not mean they are *trying* to be unhelpful; it's just an exercise in being honest about the effect other people have on you.

People encourage extreme plans

We have often discussed how extreme plans – whether eating- or activity-related – are unhelpful and often worse than no plan at all. Even if you have moved away from these approaches, it doesn't mean everyone around you has. Friends or workmates may still use them, encourage you to join them, or be openly doubtful about your approach. This is important. If friends do affect you like this, write it down.

People try to help in an unhelpful way

When other people support your plans, this can be really helpful. It can also be very annoying. Here are some examples of responses by close friends and family who are trying to help someone but probably doing the opposite:

- *Are you sure you should be eating that?*
- *You have missed your exercise class twice this week. You will never lose weight like that.*
- *You don't need to lose weight – you look fine to me.* (This was the partner of someone with a high BMI who wanted to lose some weight to help manage some health problems.)
- *Of course, if you want to exercise, you will need a decent pair of running shoes. Those ones are no good. And I can give you some good advice on training schedules. . .*

> • *I'll just make you a green salad for your evening meal – that will help, won't it?*

You can see what's happening, can't you? Most of us do not like to be monitored or have the idea that someone is checking up on us. Someone who is regularly trying to 'help' can seem like a spy with a video camera! Also, other people's advice can feel controlling and many people will rebel and do the opposite. This is understandable – but unfortunately it can ruin perfectly good plans. Again, if there are any examples like this in your life, write them down.

So far, we have covered the things that people directly *say* or *do* to you. However, there is another way, even harder to see at times, in which other people affect you: by influencing your attitudes.

Other people affect what seems 'normal'

Nobody is born knowing *what* to eat and in what quantities, or how much activity to take to stay healthy. However, most of us go through our lives thinking we know what is 'normal'. In fact, most of our ideas are learned from other people. We see what our parents ate and how active they were, and this has a strong influence on us. Later in life, friends and partners have an effect. All of this influences what we think of as 'normal' or 'usual'.

WHAT IS A 'NORMAL' LEVEL OF ACTIVITY AND EXERCISE?

To get an idea of what we mean, look at the following questions about activity.

- Is it 'normal' to take the stairs, or the lift? Is it 'normal' to walk somewhere or take the car?
- Is it 'normal' to use a bike to get around?
- Is it 'normal' to take regular exercise or to avoid it?
- Do 'most' people take active holidays such as walking or 'inactive' holidays like sitting on a beach?
- Is it 'normal' to always take a shortcut or to walk a little further?
- Is it 'normal' to accept the offer of a lift or to politely refuse because you need your walk?
- Is it 'normal' to have exercise equipment at home or to own sports clothes? Or is it 'normal' to think that people who enjoy exercise are a bit weird?
- Is it 'obvious' that running can damage your knees?

Whatever your answers to these questions, they are not 'common sense' or 'what normal people do' – they are in fact *beliefs and thoughts*, like those we discussed in chapter 2.

Most people do not spend much time questioning these beliefs – partly because they don't often question any of their beliefs and also because things may seem 'normal' when *lots of people around you are doing these things*. But just because something is the usual habit of lots of people, doesn't make it healthy.

It's a very good idea to look at what you think is 'normal' for activity and to realise these beliefs are often heavily influenced by other people and not because you consulted an expert who advised this approach.

WHAT IS A 'NORMAL' STYLE OF EATING?

The same points apply to food and eating:

* Is it 'normal' to have a dessert?
* Is it 'normal' to have breakfast?
* How many times a day do 'normal' people eat?
* How often is it 'normal' to have a snack between meals?
* How often is it 'normal' to have fast food or takeaway food?
* Is it 'normal' to crave chocolate?
* Is it 'normal' to eat late at night?
* Is it 'normal' to snack in front of the TV?
* Is it 'normal' to usually buy a snack when you go into a shop?
* Is it 'normal' to reward yourself with food?

Kirsty certainly noticed how this had an effect on her:

> *A few years ago, I was living in a shared house with friends. It had a huge effect on my habits and weight. Very often we would sit down during the evening as a group and watch a film together. When we did this, it was just normal to order pizza and have a few bowls of crisps to snack on. One day I just woke up and realised what I was doing – a couple of times a week, I was eating so much I often felt uncomfortably full. Nobody was making me eat a whole pizza and crisps whilst watching a film, but at the time, it just seemed like the thing to do – it had become a habit. I am more aware of that kind of thing now.*

Pete also had a moment when he realised what he was doing:

> *I have to travel quite a bit with my job and so do a lot of driving. In the past, whenever I stopped to get fuel or have a break I would get a snack at the same time, usually a chocolate bar. Everyone else seemed to be doing it, so I thought, why not. Of course, I realised later that other people may not be travelling as much as I do or don't always get a snack every time they stop for fuel or a break – they just do it occasionally. But I thought that buying something every time was just normal.*

Both Kirsty and Pete were being guided by thoughts and beliefs about what was 'usual/normal' and people around them seemed to support these beliefs, so it wasn't easy to question their beliefs and see them for what they were – just beliefs, not necessarily the truth.

OTHER IDEAS THAT CAN SEEM NORMAL

The final type of belief is a bit more general. It is usually an attitude towards eating or activity passed through a family or culture. Some of these may seem familiar:

- When it comes to exercise, it's a case of 'no pain, no gain'.
- You should never waste food – there are people starving in the world.
- Always clear your plate.
- It's rude to refuse the food people offer you – to be polite you must eat everything offered by your host.
- Some people are cut out for exercise and some people aren't.
- Refusing the food someone offers you is rejecting that person.
- People who are active don't know how to relax and enjoy life.
- If there's a family history of weight gain then there's nothing you can do to improve your situation – its just inevitable.
- People who turn down food are fussy and rude.

Most families have 'rules' like these and it is easy to see how these ideas can affect people's plans.

However, it's helpful to understand they are just ideas and not necessarily the 'truth'.

Check that your problem is really what you think it is

By now you will have looked at a number of ways in which other people can affect your plans. Hopefully, you have been writing things down and now have a list of areas where things are difficult. It's time to work on solutions to these problems.

To summarise, we have covered four different types of problem:

1. People change your environment in a way that makes change harder.
2. People don't give you practical support when you rely on them.
3. People encourage and discourage you.
4. People may make less-healthy eating and activity habits seem 'normal'.

This is a big range of problems and a few different ideas and skills will be needed to deal with them. However, first it is useful to ask a few questions. Earlier, we saw that people tend to presume that their view of a situation is the truth and seldom spend much time checking whether they are right. It is worth checking that your view of your problem situation(s) is completely accurate. If there are other, more helpful ways of seeing a situation, it's worth spending time on finding them. Things that seem like a serious block could look very different from another angle. You could use the question and expand skills from chapter 2 for this. Here we have focused on a few key issues.

Check your facts

It's obviously important to check your facts when it comes to a belief about 'normal' eating and activity. How would you know? How many 'normal' people have you asked? Have you asked a medical or nutrition expert, for example? And even if you do come to the conclusion that your habit or belief is normal, is it healthy?

Check your facts too when it comes to your 'problem' situations. For example, if you have identified a way in which someone does not give you important practical help, is it really impossible to do what you want to do without their help? Have you really thought through all of the ways in which you might manage on your own? If you have not gone through some systematic problem-solving on this issue (*see chapter 6*) then you do not actually know what you might be able to manage on your own.

Similarly, if other people's discouragement – or encouragement – is blocking you, is it really true that if they went away one day things would be perfect? Have they always ruined your plans or have there been other times when you have stuck to your guns? If you have, is the current situation really all their fault?

It's always easy to blame other people. However, the truth is often more complicated. The purpose of 'checking your facts' is not to blame *you* for everything or to make you feel guilty. However, if the problem lies partly with you as well as with others, then this is actually *good* news. You have more control over yourself than you have over other people. It means that you can start to change right now, by working on your own habits.

Be open about mixed feelings

For example, many people have their plans spoiled by others encouraging them to eat more than they had planned. Whether it is a grandmother serving an extra-large portion or friends buying a dessert, this can be a problem. However, when you're in this situation would you be completely unhappy or would part of you be quite pleased?

It can be very useful to be open about mixed feelings like this. Once you start to be honest with yourself, you can start to think about what you really want – in the long term, as well as the short term. You can make clear decisions about what's most important for you.

Check you have really told people what you want

As we discussed above, it's easy to think other people are to blame for not helping. However, are you sure you have really asked the people involved to start helping – or to stop what they are doing? Think about this seriously. Have you asked them in a really direct, clear way (*see SMART, chapter 6*) what you want them to do?

If you want to check for yourself, think about the last time you raised the issue. Write it down or imagine it from the other person's perspective. Imagine they were a little tired or distracted when they heard it. Imagine they did not really think it mattered much to you. Did you manage to express yourself in a way that was completely clear and impossible to get wrong?

Let's look now at how to communicate in a way that is clear, respectful and effective.

Deal with the people involved – raise the issue and negotiate

You may have decided – after checking your facts – that there really is a problem with another person. Something they are doing is getting in the way of your plans. If this is the case you need to ask them to behave differently. It may sound simple, but it often feels difficult to do. Imagine saying to your friends: 'Please could you stop suggesting we go for chips on a night out. Instead, please could you accompany me to a salad bar?' You probably wouldn't get very far. . .

There are a couple of important truths about dealing with other people. First, it is clear you will not be able to control anyone else's behaviour. People will do what they like, and you cannot directly change that. However, you *can* change the way you communicate with them. You can seriously influence how likely a person is to listen to you by how you approach them and what you say.

Usually, people do not handle these difficult conversations very well. They tend to do one (or more) of four things:

1. Avoid the issue and not mention it at all.
2. Raise the issue, but then give in as soon as the other person disagrees.
3. Get angry with the other person.
4. Grumble, mutter, be sarcastic or try to give the person hints about what they should be doing.

Pete has tried all of the above.

> *Ann often buys in food that I just can't resist. I hate it when there's lots of ice cream in the freezer. Of course, part of me loves it too and I really don't seem to be able to resist eating lots of it when it's around. I haven't really talked to Ann about it – apart from last night. Generally, I just avoid the topic. I've tried to drop some hints – not very clever really, I'd just say something like 'Oh, ice cream again – that's nice and healthy!' She never seemed to get the message, but I guess that's not surprising. I got more and more fed up about the situation. Finally, last night, I flipped – started yelling at her, telling her she should be more considerate and try to help me, and not*

sabotage my plans. It was awful. I made her cry and I feel like a horrible person.

Kirsty has had no more luck:

I often go out for a drink on a Friday with my work buddy Celia. She's great fun and we have a good time. However, there's always a point in the evening when she says, 'Let's go for a pizza!' I know Celia well – when she has got her mind on something, nothing is likely to change it. I usually just groan to myself and go to the pizza place, promising my healthy-eating plan can start again next week. I have tried to persuade her to go somewhere else, but she says, 'That's boring! Let's go for a pizza!' and I never know what to say. I just end up following her.

None of Pete or Kirsty's efforts have gone very well so far. However, these conversations are not easy. You need to do many things at once – stick to your guns and get your point across whilst being calm and respectful towards the other person. You also need to be very clear and able to talk about how the situation makes you feel. There is quite a lot to think about, so we will take it a step at a time. The first step is to clear your head.

Clear your head

Before you start having your difficult conversation, you need to check your view of the situation is not going to get in the way. Using the skills from chapter 2, catch your thoughts about the situation. Pinpoint them, explain and summarise them. Watch out for thoughts about the other person ('They are doing it on purpose!' 'They don't care!') and about what is fair and unfair in the situation ('How dare they!'). Here are some examples from Pete and Kirsty's situations:

> **Pete:** *My main thought is, 'She's so inconsiderate!' There is also, 'She doesn't care about my health' and 'She doesn't listen to me'.*

> **Kirsty:** *It's something like, 'There's no point, she won't listen.' Also, some thoughts about her: 'She's just a good-time girl, she won't really care, and she'll probably think I'm boring.'*

Remember, these thoughts may be untrue or unhelpful. We often make assumptions about other people even though we know nothing about how they feel or how they see things. We also never know exactly how our own behaviour looks to others and how it might affect them.

So, notice your thoughts and then put them to one side. You might be right, but you might not. You do not know the other person's side of the story. Your judgement may be wrong. Focus on the things they are *doing* that are causing you problems, rather than on your opinion of their *character*.

The second part of 'clearing your head' is becoming clear about what you want to get out of the conversation. You need to think this through in advance. The authors of a help-ful book on this topic, *Difficult Conversations* (*see Appendix II*), imagine what it would be like if NASA scientists were to say: 'Well, we'll just launch the rocket up towards space and see what happens – we'll take it from there.' This may sound obviously impractical, but many people do start off their difficult conversations like this.

If you want another person to do something differently, you must be prepared to give them a clear example of what you would like them to do. For example, does Pete really want Ann never to buy ice cream again under any circum-stances? Even if they have guests or on special occasions? He needs to think this through in advance. If he can't tell Ann how he wants things to be different, then he cannot complain if she doesn't get it right. It can help to use the SMART principle here (see page 216). Be prepared to give the other person some Specific, Measurable examples of how you would like them to change, ideas they have some chance of Agreeing to, and that are Realistic and on a Timetable.

Pick your moment – then start talking about the situation 'from above'

PICK YOUR MOMENT

When you have some idea of what you want to achieve, you can think about raising the topic. Only you can decide when it is a good time to start a difficult conversation, but here are a few guidelines:

- Try to leave yourself plenty of time for the conversation.
- Try to pick a time when neither of you is too stressed.
- Don't 'ambush' the other person – the idea is to have a real conversation with them rather than to force them to agree with you quickly or embarrass them in front of others.

There is probably never a perfect moment for some conversations – just try to pick a relatively good one.

TALK 'FROM ABOVE'

The next principle is to start to talk about the situation 'from above' – as if you were seeing the other person's behaviour *and* your own behaviour from the outside. This is important because when we are not happy with another person's behaviour we can usually only see our side of the story. However, this is no way to start a conversation. Imagine if a friend came up to you and said: 'I don't know why you are being so inconsiderate! What you are doing is so hurtful that you really have no excuse. . .' Would you really feel like listening to the rest of what they had to say? So, step away from your personal point of view and talk about the situation as if you were an observer.

Here are some good rules for starting the conversation:

- Talk about the situation as if you were observing it from the outside.
- Talk about facts and behaviour, rather than your opinion of the other person's character.
- Make it clear this is your point of view – and that you might have got it wrong.
- Say something positive about the other person and acknowledge you have also contributed to the problem.
- Talk about yourself and how you feel, rather than judging the other person's behaviour and character.

Pete is doing a great job of using these ideas:

'Ann, I have been thinking about the food we buy for the house. I know you do all the shopping – it's a lot of work and I really appreciate you organising it. However, as you know I'm trying to change my eating habits, but I find it really, really hard to resist ice cream when it's in the freezer. It would be very helpful if we could avoid having it in the house – or at least just have it in once in a while. It would make a lot of difference to me. I know in an ideal world I would just be able to avoid eating it regularly but that doesn't seem to work at the moment. I'd really appreciate it if we could change what we buy – it would mean a lot to me and help me out. What do you think?'

Here Pete is speaking 'from above' as an observer and then speaking clearly about what he wants.

The next example shows how he might do it if he were ignoring these guidelines:

> '*Ann, I have been thinking about the food we buy for the house. It's really annoying me. I need you to start thinking a bit more about my needs. You know I really struggle with ice cream when it's in the house, but you carry on buying it. I'm not quite sure what your problem is, but you need to get this clear in your head: no more ice cream – OK?*'

In this situation, Pete is being calm and stating what he wants, but he is not saying it in a way that Ann is likely to be interested in listening to. Ask yourself if you honestly respond well when people speak to you in this way. Also, which approach will start a conversation? Which will encourage Ann to speak to Pete and perhaps even tell him things about his own behaviour that he does not realise?

Ask for help and listen to what the other person has to say

The idea is to start a useful conversation and to state your own wishes clearly and directly. This will not only produce better long-term relationships but also have a number of immediate benefits. It makes the other person feel you value their opinion and are interested in what they have to say. This will make them more likely to respond positively. Also, you are more likely to learn something. Remember, the other person may have information that can help you.

You may notice that Pete ended by saying, 'What do you think?' By doing this, he is inviting Ann to get involved in the discussion. He is saying to her – though not out loud – 'I care what you think, and I would appreciate your opinion and help.' This is a good first step. However, the next step is more important: you must be genuinely willing to listen to what the other person has to say. This means being prepared to consider changing your view about a situation. This is important. If you listen but do not really hear, then you will learn nothing. Also, the other person will notice.

Here are a few quick rules about what other people can tell about you in difficult conversations:

- They can tell when you are not really listening to them.
- They can tell when they are being pushed into something.
- They can tell when you have already made up your mind about something and are not seriously considering any other alternative.

However, if you are genuine, then people are likely to tell you their point of view and help out.

Pete decided to grit his teeth and really listen to what Ann had to say:

> *Ann: I really didn't think that it mattered that much. I mean, whenever we have ice cream in the house, you eat it! I thought that meant you liked it. . .*
>
> *Pete: But you know I'm trying to change my eating habits and lose weight. And I don't exactly look pleased when I see you have bought some, do I?*
>
> *Ann: Sure. Of course, I noticed you looking a bit grumpy. Then you would usually start eating it! I thought, 'If it really matters, he'll say something.' And you never did. Until now.*
>
> *Pete: Oh.*
>
> *Ann: I'm not really that keen on ice cream. It's usually you that finishes the carton. I don't mind not getting it.*

Pete has probably learned something from this conversation. It is clear that relying on Ann to 'guess' how he feels about food isn't good enough. Also, this conversation showed him his thoughts about the situation – that Ann was inconsiderate and didn't listen – were completely wide of the mark. She was paying close attention to his behaviour all along. However, he was not communicating clearly.

Of course, difficult conversations do not always go as well as this. They are usually a lot more tense. In the situation above, Pete is not asking Ann to make much of a sacrifice, as she doesn't really like ice cream. When the other person feels they do have to sacrifice something, they will sometimes try to resist you. This can take a few different forms, such as:

- Ignoring you
- Treating what you say as unimportant
- Changing the subject
- Making it all into a joke
- Implying you are being selfish
- Giving lots of reasons (excuses) why they can't do it
- Saying they didn't mean to be unhelpful (and therefore that their behaviour is OK)
- Arguing
- Simply refusing altogether

All of these things are difficult to deal with. Most of us hate getting into arguments. Also, it's easy to start thinking you have got it wrong when the other person is being forceful or persuasive. In these situations, some extra techniques are needed.

Talk about yourself clearly and forcefully

Kirsty's friend Celia is a bit more of a handful than Ann. Here is Kirsty's first attempt to talk to her:

Kirsty: Listen, Celia, I know we usually go for pizza at this point in the evening, but I'd really rather try something a bit more healthy. Instead, we could go to—

Celia: [cutting in] Come on, you know you want to! [laughs]

Kirsty: But maybe this time we could—

Celia: [cutting in again] Oh come on, girl, it's getting late! Friday night is pizza night. Get your coat.

Kirsty: [speechless] . . . [gets her coat]

It took Kirsty quite a while to get up the courage to have this conversation and afterwards she felt hopeless about the whole thing. She wondered how she would ever manage when Celia would not even let her finish her sentences.

In situations like this:

1. Talk about yourself and your feelings.
2. Be very clear and concrete about what you want to happen.
3. If you get into a discussion or negotiation, be clear what your 'bottom line' is, so you don't end up agreeing to something you feel uncomfortable with.
4. Repeat yourself. State your point of view again. And again. And again. (The 'broken record' technique.)

Here is Kirsty putting these ideas into action:

Celia: OK, it's time for some food! Let's go.

314

Kirsty: Seriously, Celia, this evening I want to go somewhere other than the pizza place.

Celia: Oh, come on, Kirsty, you know we always go for a pizza!

Kirsty: I know we have in the past, but—

Celia: [cutting in] It's getting late, let's go.

Kirsty: Celia, this matters to me and I need you to listen to me now. I would like to go for some food that is healthier than pizza.

Celia: This is all about your weight, isn't it? I wish you would just accept that you are a beautiful woman the way you are.

Kirsty: Thanks, Celia, but it's about my health as well, and my health matters to me. I would like to go somewhere different this evening.

Celia: God, you're really hung up on this, aren't you?

Kirsty: This is important to me. I'd like to go somewhere else.

Celia: OK, let's go some other place next time. . .

Kirsty: No, I would like to try somewhere else this evening.

Celia: All right, all right! You're kind of scary this evening! I give in. Do you have somewhere in mind?

Here Kirsty has used the 'broken record' technique very

OVERCOMING WEIGHT PROBLEMS

well. She said that she wanted to go to a different place *five times*. Eventually, Celia realised that she would say it twenty-five times if necessary and decided that she had better listen. This is the beauty of the 'broken record' technique. It makes it clear to other people that you will say the same thing no matter how they try to distract you or argue with you.

The second important point is that Kirsty just talked about herself – she mentioned what was important *to her* and what *she* wanted. She did not get into a conversation about how Celia wasn't listening or helping. It is important not to start accusing other people or labelling their behaviour as unhelpful. Here are the reasons for this:

- Whilst you are talking about yourself – what matters to you and what you want to happen – you can only be right. Nobody knows you better than you do, so it makes it hard for the other person to argue.
- On the other hand, if you start accusing the other person and labelling their behaviour and their character, they can (sometimes with reason) disagree and start an argument. You are no longer on solid ground. Also, you will offend people and make them less likely to listen to you.

There are, however, some mistakes that you can make when talking about yourself.

For example: 'I've been feeling that you're very selfish and you never listen' This may be direct and open and momentarily you may feel you've got things off your chest, but it isn't a smart move. Imagine how this feels from the other person's perspective. Would you get the impression they wanted to start a constructive conversation? Would you be more or less likely to make an effort for them?

So, when you're trying to have a difficult conversation, you need to talk clearly about yourself, but you also need to watch out for any urges to tell people what you really think of them as it's likely to ruin your chances of managing the conversation well.

Here's another way of managing the same statement:

> *I have been getting upset and I've been finding it hard to know what to think. From my point of view, I have tried to raise this issue with you a few times. However, I don't think we have ever had a good talk about it, and I have never seen you suggest a way you can help. You are generally the kind of person who's happy to help with something like this. Perhaps I have not been making clear how much this matters to me. It really does matter to me. Can we talk about it right now?*

How would you feel this time if someone said that to you?

Difficult conversations are just that – difficult. You have to have several different things in your head. For example, you must be willing to negotiate, but have an idea about your 'bottom line' and be willing to stick to it. It's hard.

You can explore this topic more by looking at some of the books in Appendix II. But in the meantime it's worth practising the skills. If you wait until you feel confident before having a go, you may wait for ever.

However, there is one other big block that stops people from getting started:

FEELING GUILTY AND SELFISH IN DIFFICULT CONVERSATIONS

If you are having a difficult conversation, this usually means you are talking about things that are important to you and are asking other people to change their behaviour in some way. This often triggers thoughts like:

I'm being selfish.

I shouldn't put myself first – I should be thinking of others more.

They will think that I'm a really pushy person.

If this happens, use your skills from chapter 2. Look at the thoughts and beliefs that flicker through your head when you are having these conversations or when you're thinking about them. These thoughts are just thoughts and are not necessarily true or helpful. Use your question and expand skills here.

When you are having a difficult conversation, you're not doing anything very radical. All you are doing is saying something about yourself and your health. It is something you have thought hard about, and you have decided is important to you. You are just asking the other person to listen while you tell them about a way in which they could help. You are willing to listen to their point of view. You are not yelling or saying things about their character. So *how can doing this be selfish?* The answer of course is that it's not selfish, it is just clear communication about something important. If the other person thinks it's selfish, then that's their problem, not yours.

Many people think they should consider others' needs and try to put other people first, and there is a place for this sometimes when being kind and considerate. However, if you are considerate and listen to other people, then you too have the right to be listened to and shown consideration. Your needs are as important as anyone else's. And the more you look after your own health and emotional wellbeing, the better you will be able to care for others.

Make your own plan

Unfortunately, having a well-planned and well-managed difficult conversation does not guarantee you will get the results you want. It makes getting what you want more likely, but sometimes people will still ignore your needs, and there are some other people you will simply not be able to negotiate with at all.

If you get into trouble with your difficult conversations, you will probably be having one (or both) of two difficulties:

1. You are not getting practical help from the other person.
2. The other person is being discouraging or abusive.

We discussed practical support above. Abuse can take a few different forms. Here are some examples:

- Open verbal abuse such as name calling
- Scorn and contempt
- Teasing
- Undermining you and saying negative things about what you are capable of

These can be very upsetting and destructive and can certainly spoil someone's planned changes.

There are two steps for dealing with these issues. The first is to think practically.

Try to sort things out on your own

This is the obvious first step when you are not getting the support you need. If this is your problem, try thinking about the issues using your problem-solving skills from chapter 6. For example:

- If you need your partner to look after someone you care for whilst you get some exercise, could someone else cover for you?

- If there's no one to look after your kids while you exercise, could you find an activity you could all do together?
- If your family insist on buying less-healthy snacks you find tempting, could you put them in an out-of-reach cupboard?
- If your friend often gives you food gifts like chocolates, could you give them to someone else or donate them to a raffle?

Obviously, there are no simple solutions to the difficulties you listed, or you would not have listed them. But remember, you never know how close a solution is until you start looking for it!

It is also a good idea to start with practical solutions when other people are being negative or abusive. For example, when **Sandra** goes for a walk some of the local kids say unkind things. There may be practical options here, for example:

- Are the kids there all the time? Could she go out when they are usually away?
- Is there some way of checking whether they are there or not before going out?
- Are there any other routes she could take?
- Could she go out once or twice with a friend?

It is always worth checking you have covered all of the practical options. However, even good problem-solving does not guarantee an answer. You may still be left in a situation in which people are negative or abusive and spoiling your plans. You may not be able to change the abuse, but you can change how you respond to it.

Take a different view

Many people come across rudeness and abuse in their lives. Some of the time this really hurts and some of the time it's not too bad. The type of abuse matters, and some people are more able to hurt us than others. Also, it depends on how we are feeling on that particular day – some days we can shrug things off and some days everything hurts. A lot depends on how we see the situation – in other words, what we think about the situation at the time. If we change our thinking, we can change how the situation affects us.

The thoughts in Sandra's head went something like this:

> *I thought if I went out during the day, no one would see me . . . They are so cruel, just picking on anyone who looks different . . . I just can't handle these unpleasant comments on a daily basis . . . How dare they? How do they have the right to treat me like this?*

There are a few different types of thought here: thoughts about the other people and thoughts about Sandra herself and her ability to cope. When we are upset by abuse, our thinking often runs along these lines.

If you have a situation similar to Sandra's that is making you upset, use your skills from chapter 2 and pinpoint the thoughts. Try to summarise what is most upsetting about the situation. You already know the procedure for dealing with these thoughts. You can get going right now, using your question and expand skills. Below are some questions that can help you:

- **Questions about the other people:**

  Why are they doing this?

  What might have happened or be happening in their lives to explain why they are behaving in this way?

  Do they really understand my situation?

  Why don't they have anything better to do with their time?

  Why do they feel so uncomfortable about me?

  How do they have the right to judge me?

  If I decide not to be affected by these people, are they really able to hurt me? If I decide to ignore their words, how much can they hurt me?

OVERCOMING WEIGHT PROBLEMS

- **Questions about yourself and your ability to cope:**

  Why do I have to meet some kind of standard or be some particular way to be acceptable? Why do I have to 'pass' someone else's 'test' to be OK?

  What does my size have to do with my character or my quality as a person?

  Don't I have a right to do what I like, walk where I like? If they don't like it, they don't have to pay any attention to it.

  Do I want to let these people spoil the quality of my day? Do I want to let them spoil my plans?

  How many other unkind people have I dealt with in my life? If I have dealt with them, why can't I deal with this lot?

  Do I know anyone else – either personally or a fictional character – who has put up with a lot of unkindness but kept going and kept their pride? What can I learn from them?

Sandra went through this process and ended up feeling a little differently about her situation:

I ended up thinking of the local kids as just silly, annoying children who had no understanding of my life.

And although they were annoying they weren't worth getting upset over! I noticed they only do it in a group. Whenever I pass one of the kids on their own, they don't say a thing. That says a lot about why they are doing it and about how brave they are. . . One of my neighbours told me that a couple of the kids have really tough home lives so maybe that's part of why they want to be cruel to me; it makes them feel better about themselves. When I stopped to think what might make them do this it helped me see the problem was with them and not with me. I guess I also got a bit of my pride back and held my head up a bit more. I still do practical things – I still try to go out when they are least likely to be around! – but I have taken a serious decision about whether I will let them stop me doing what I want. Fourteen-year-olds are not going to get in the way of my plans.

In Sandra's case, the problem did not go away, but changing her attitude towards it improved both her feelings and her ability to get on with her plans.

However, even if a person changes their thinking about a situation, this may not completely take away the shame, sadness or anger they feel when another person treats them badly. So, it is useful to decide what to do with these emotions.

Are you willing to tolerate unpleasant feelings?

Difficult situations create unpleasant feelings. Look at Sandra's situation. She felt embarrassed, humiliated, angry, upset and ashamed. What would have happened if she had decided these feelings were so awful she couldn't accept them under any circumstances? She would never have left her house again. Unfortunately, it is true other people can cause us unpleasant feelings and they sometimes decide to do so on purpose. There's not a lot we can do about this. But how we treat the feelings can make a huge difference. The whole issue can be summed up in one sentence:

> *So long as you try to avoid the unpleasant feelings that other people can cause you, then they control you.*

For example, if you never want to feel upset and angry, then you will never confront another person about an issue – and that means it is very unlikely to change. If you never want to feel embarrassed, then you will probably never try to learn something new, try out a new activity in public – and this means your thoughts about other people are controlling your behaviour, rather than your own plans.

On the other hand, the opposite is also true:

> *The moment you decide you can put up with the unpleasant feelings you may feel in response to other people, they no longer have any control over you.*

If you decide you will raise an issue with someone, even

though it will make you tense and angry, then you are in charge. If you decide you will go swimming, even though you feel embarrassed in a swimsuit, then you are in charge. This is a bit like the exercises in 'holding steady' in chapter 7 (page 277). You will not be able to get rid of bad feelings altogether, but you can change how you treat them. Emotions are not as powerful and unbearable as they feel – and when you decide to accept them and experience them anyway, they often lose their power.

CHAPTER SUMMARY

- Check how other people affect you – both in practical ways and in how they treat you.
- Don't take your view of the situation as the automatic truth – check it first.
- Raise difficult issues with people when you can – but think about when to do it and how to do it skilfully.
- If this doesn't work – or if there are people you can't negotiate with – find ways to carry out your plans anyway.
- Your reasons for managing weight are important and you can find ways to move towards them with or without other people's help.

9

Keeping it going

I've made some great changes so far. Let's hope they last.

I think I've been here before – I've been given lots of good ideas and then left to keep going – for the rest of my life, on my own!

This book started by pointing out that changing eating and activity habits and managing weight in the long term is difficult. It is. This is because you need to make changes *and then keep those changes going*. Managing weight is more like a distance race than a sprint and your plan needs to 'go the distance'.

Over time a lot of things can change in people's lives. Jobs, relationships, moods – and you need a plan that will see you through all of these. Everyone experiences setbacks and comes across challenges when they make changes to their habits. Here are a few examples:

> • You might slip with your plans but hardly notice it, then suddenly realise you have gained quite a lot of weight.

- You may get stuck and feel as though there's nothing you can do.
- You may find yourself going backwards.
- It may be hard to know when to keep going and when to be happy with what you have achieved.
- After trying for some time, you may realise you are dealing with a serious problem with your emotions.

Don't panic – you can actively work through all of these difficulties. This chapter will give you practical, positive ways of doing so. It will also cover the scientific research on why people find it difficult to keep going with their plans.

How to stop things just slipping away

It is easy to stop thinking about something without even noticing you have stopped. For example, most people have had the sudden realisation they have forgotten something – an unpaid bill, a friend's birthday – for a very long time. The same can happen when changing habits and managing weight – eating and activity habits can slowly slide and then suddenly you realise you've gained weight.

Losing awareness and focus like this is very common. Although most people can think of areas in their life where they do keep focused on a goal for long periods, for example studying for an academic qualification for years, there are usually other people such as tutors helping them keep on track.

However, eating and activity changes can start slipping away, particularly after you've gone past the first few months and if you don't have help from other people or any external goals to keep you focused.

Clearly, you are more likely to keep going if you have a plan for long-term change. Just deciding you will 'try to remember to keep on track' will probably not be good enough. There are two useful steps that can help here. The first is to look at any mixed feelings you may have about carrying on with your weight-change plan. Second, there are some practical ideas that can help.

Check your thoughts about the long term

Many people find thinking about food and activity changes as long-term rather difficult. As with most mixed feelings, it is best to be clear about this. Stop for a moment and imagine having to keep an eye on eating and activity for the next five years of your life. Try to pinpoint (chapter 2) the emotions and the thoughts that go along with this idea. You may find some thoughts like:

It's all such a huge effort.

Five years without being able to relax. . . This is miserable – where's the fun?

It will be a process of starving and restricting myself. No way. You can't make me do it. I'll do what I like.

Try to pinpoint your own personal thoughts about this. Then you can use your question and expand skills to check if these thoughts are really true and helpful. Taking the examples above, how much effort are we talking about exactly? And maybe you do want to relax, but are you relaxed right now about your weight? How relaxed would you be if your health got worse? Very often, people think of the need for continued food and activity changes as someone trying to control them or spoil their fun. Is this really the case? And don't you have your own important reasons for managing weight?

Remember, the aim is to make sensible, reasonable plans that you can imagine sticking to for the long term. These plans should not be extreme or restrictive. And ultimately, being healthy may be just as much fun as overeating or being inactive, if not more so!

If you spend a couple of minutes with your notebook looking at your thoughts and seeing how balanced they are, it will be time very well spent.

Make some appointments

Once you have considered carefully any mixed feelings you may have, you will have a better chance of success with your plan. However, you will still need a prompt once in a while to check you have not lost track of where you are. Reminders are always helpful.

So, you need to make some appointments. The first type of appointment is to carve out some quality time when you can think about your own health undisturbed. Maybe have a particular day/time once a month to check on your progress. If you wish, you can use the space to do some problem-solving about issues that are proving difficult.

Some people use diaries or a calendar to make this work whereas others just pick memorable dates.

Here's how **Sandra** made this work:

> *I have never used a diary and I'm not about to start now. So, to make some time to think through my progress over the next six months, I've decided to set some time aside at Easter, then the day after Don's birthday and finally before our summer holiday. Three appointments, no diary.*

Booking time with other people can also be helpful. This may be your family doctor or nurse if there is a particular medical issue linked with your weight or if you wish to discuss progress with managing weight. A commercial weight-management group or friends can also provide support. Whoever you choose, make sure it is someone who will be friendly and supportive. This is not meant to be a check on whether you have been 'good' or not. It's meant to be a way of keeping track and checking in with yourself.

As mentioned in previous chapters, digital technology such as apps and wearable devices can really help with motivation and keeping on track. There is more information about this in the appendices.

Getting stuck and going backwards

As well as having plans to keep focused it is also important to think about how you are going to respond when things go wrong. For the majority of people, once in a while, even with good plans, things will still go wrong, and you may get stuck.

Responses

Getting stuck – when nothing is working, and you can't see a way forward – can be upsetting. It can lead to feeling hopeless, frustrated and can sometimes result in weight gain.

Generally, when things go wrong two things happen. First, you have thoughts about the situation. Your mind will certainly have a view on what is happening and what that means about you, managing your weight and the future (and it probably won't be very positive). Second, you will react on the basis of these thoughts.

What you actually do at this point can be more helpful or less helpful. The following will be very unhelpful:

- Giving up. Starting eating and exercising according to old habits
- Deciding to stop trying for a while – a week, a month, a year. . .
- Trying very hard not to think about the whole issue of weight and health

- Feeling miserable and doing nothing
- Searching for new magic cures or new medical opinions
- Blaming someone else and avoiding any habit adjustments 'until the other person changes'
- Going back to using extreme or fad diets which are unlikely to help

All of these reactions are very understandable – they make perfect sense, given the circumstances – but they won't get you anywhere.

Research shows why some of these reactions are unhelpful. In women who had taken part in a CBT weight-management programme and recorded when they were tempted to give up and the times they actually did, the number of times they felt like throwing in the towel did not seem to matter. The only important factor seemed to be *their response to the temptation*. Those who believed a minor setback was a disaster failed the most. When some kind of 'coping' response was used participants kept themselves on track. There were many different types of helpful coping approaches and the main message of this research was the power to keep on track is inside you – by thinking differently about setbacks and finding ways to cope.

Here are some ideas on how to cope well.

A positive response

It's important to be realistic here. The first step in dealing with a setback is to accept it is happening. If it is a serious setback, then it is definitely worth being open about it.

Recall the two main responses to setbacks: thoughts about the situation and then actions. Both of these need to be managed.

THINK AHEAD

First, it's a good idea to decide in advance how you are going to think about such situations. **Pete** decided to use the idea of managing his weight and health as a distance race:

> *The way I see it, improving my health is going to take a long time. It's like a distance race – kind of like a marathon. If you watch marathon runners, you see they aren't bothered if one of their opponents goes in front. They know there is plenty of time to make up the gap – or for their opponent to become tired. They don't panic, think they are going to lose and change their plans. I'm going to keep going with my eating and activity plans. I'll get there in the end, even with a couple of slips on the way.*

Have a think about how you would like to approach setbacks. If you work this out in advance, you are more likely to cope well. Some people use sayings like 'Two steps forward, one step back' or 'Don't make a mountain out of a molehill.' See what you think might work for you. Anything will do,

335

OVERCOMING WEIGHT PROBLEMS

so long as it makes sense and will allow you to be calm and practical when things get difficult. Again, if you spend a few minutes with your notebook thinking about this *right now*, it will really help in the long term.

MAKE THE RIGHT MOVES

Second, it is critical to make the right moves when things are not going to plan. People often run into problems with this.

1. They get stuck in how awful it is, lose focus on doing practical things to help themselves, or hope someone else will fix it for them.
2. They start using plans that are extreme diets or unlikely to help.

During difficult times it's really important to remember to use your CBT skills rather than thinking they aren't working. Experiencing setbacks doesn't mean CBT has failed, it just means life is throwing something difficult at you. CBT is a set of tools or skills and when setbacks occur it's a chance to learn from these experiences and refine your skills so the next time this happens you'll hopefully be in a better place to deal with things differently.

So, when you're getting stuck or in a difficult place you might:

- Do some problem-solving.
- Check your reasons and your motivation are clear and strong.
- See if any thoughts or beliefs are getting in your way.
- Remind yourself that lapses are normal and can be an opportunity to learn how to do things differently next time.
- Check you're not blaming yourself.
- Record your own behaviour to check you are not missing anything.
- Check you're eating regularly and not missing meals.
- Make some new SMART plans.
- Check if any feelings – or other people – are getting in your way.
- Ask for help from understanding friends, relatives or health professionals.

Problem-solving is probably the most useful technique in dealing with setbacks and, as we noted in chapter 6, there is scientific evidence suggesting regular formal problem-solving can help keep weight off. However, there is one final thing you might need to do:

Check your facts

It is very easy to become confused about the most helpful eating and activity changes to manage weight and health, particularly given the amount of misinformation in the general media.

Sometimes people make food and activity changes believing they are genuinely going to help them achieve their goals, but if they've been misguided or misinformed the opposite may occur. Sometimes it's hard to know whether you're on the right track so it may be wise to get some expert advice. It's important to choose your expert wisely though, and some guidance on who to consult is provided in the appendices and later in this chapter.

Keeping it going – and knowing when to stop

So far, we have only covered the negative things you might encounter. However, at some point you may find yourself doing well and this can bring its own challenges. For example, you've lost weight, it's slowing down a bit and you've reached a decision point: 'Should I keep going or stay where I am and be happy with my progress so far?'

For many people, the answer to this question seems easy: they will stop when they have reached their 'goal weight' and not before. Many people have thought about their 'goal weight', or their 'ideal weight', for some time. Some have very strong dreams and fantasies about what they will do when they reach this weight. It can become a strong drive for wanting to continue pursuing weight loss.

Although in some instances monitoring the amount of weight lost can be helpful, it can also have some downsides. First, it is hard to know whether your goal weight is realistic – although as discussed at the beginning of the book, health improvements are usually seen with losses of 5–10kg (approximately 11–22lb).

Second, focusing on numbers alone disconnects you from the *reasons* why you want to manage weight in the first place – the reasons you worked out in chapter 1.

How do you know if your goal weight is realistic?

Another way of putting this question is: How do you know how much weight you can lose?

The answer, of course, is you don't know – no one does. There is no way of predicting what you can do. Someone once asked the Olympic sprinter Michael Johnson how fast he thought he could run. Johnson replied that he had no idea and he would only know this when he had run all of his races. He refused to guess how much he could achieve – and by doing this he avoided placing any limitations on himself. It is a wise approach.

There are two important facts to bear in mind when considering how much you might be able to lose. They come from the US National Weight Control Registry (NWCR) and CBT studies.

In the NWCR registry there are people who lose very large amounts of weight, and keep it off, by themselves without any drugs or surgery. They are not necessarily typical of most people, but it is important to recognise there are individuals who can do this.

However, the average person taking part in CBT research loses about 10 per cent of their weight, usually 5–10kg (approximately 11–22lb). Losing this amount of weight is more common. It's important to recognise this is the average loss, some people will lose more and some less. Losing this amount of weight is known to have important health benefits.

To summarise: *It is possible to lose large amounts of weight and keep it off. However, most people do not manage these large weight losses, even with professional help.*

It's important to bear *both* of these facts in mind when thinking about managing your weight. This is why goal weights can be problematic. They can be over-ambitious – or under-ambitious – and you would never know if they were. Take a look at these two people:

- One person loses 5 per cent of their body weight quite easily and then immediately stops. They say, 'I have lost as much as most people in CBT studies. This is the best people can do with professional help. Therefore, it's pointless for me to try to lose more.'
- The second person loses 15 per cent of their body weight but still doesn't get down to their fantasy weight and back into wearing the clothes they wore when they were younger. They are bitterly disappointed and become miserable.

Having a goal weight has tripped up both of these people. The first person has limited themselves unnecessarily, while the second is ignoring their progress.

It is also noticeable that goal weights are often very ambitious. Research has shown goal weights are frequently so low they are unlikely to be achieved unless some additional treatment like bariatric surgery takes place. For these reasons we are sceptical about the value of goal weights.

However, another factor to consider when deciding on how helpful measuring progress in numbers will be is to think about how this goal number on the scale relates to your specific reasons for wanting to improve health and manage weight from chapter 1. These reasons are often the most helpful way to measure progress.

Measure your progress by looking at your reasons

If a person is changing eating and activity habits and managing weight for their own important reasons – for example, to keep healthy so they can do more with their children – will they be concerned if they are not hitting a certain number on the scales but they are achieving a better-quality diet, improved fitness, and are getting to do more with their kids? In other words, which matters more – getting near to a number or achieving something important to you?

When you ask yourself whether to keep going with your changes, you can help find the answer by looking at your reasons. The real question is *not* 'Have I reached my goal weight?' but 'Have I made good progress in doing what I set out to do, for my own important reasons?'

Remember **Jackie** was hoping to get back to her job in nursing? She was also going to have more time to herself as her son became a teenager. She listed the following reasons for changing her habits:

1. To be in charge of her life in this area.
2. To safeguard her health by lowering her risk of diabetes.
3. To make sure she can keep up physically with her family on walking holidays.
4. To get into better shape to feel more comfortable in a senior nursing role.

Jackie made good progress in achieving change in these areas. She became fitter and lost weight – although not quite as much as she would have liked. Then things plateaued, weight loss stopped, and she began to doubt whether she had the real motivation to keep going:

> *I realised I had done really well in terms of my reasons. I had taken charge of things and I was tracking my diabetes risk. When my family doctor repeated my HbA1c measure [indicator of average blood-sugar level over last 2–3 months] it had fallen into the lower-risk category. I was much more active with lots of walking, in fact I think I walk more than Craig or John – they will have a hard time keeping up with me on our next holiday!*

I have so much more energy, feel less tired and this really matters from a nursing point of view. Although physically I probably won't have to do as much active work as I did when I was less experienced I'll feel better about leading a team of nurses. To be completely honest, I hadn't lost as much weight as I would have liked but deep down I knew I had done what was needed.

Jackie had made lots of progress and achieved many of the really important reasons she had thought through at the beginning of the process. She hadn't lost as much weight as she had wished for, but she was probably at her *best* weight – a weight at which she felt comfortable – and she could realistically maintain the new habits she had put in place. She decided to stop focusing on impossibly idealised body images from the media that just made her feel bad and instead focus on doing things that made her happy – things that she had put off for years, thinking they were only possible when she had reached her 'thin' ideal.

People's reasons for wanting to change habits and weight are not usually concrete goals that once achieved don't need to be maintained. For example, 'getting fit so I can keep up with the kids' is not something that once achieved can be discontinued without an adverse effect on the initial reason. One of Jackie's reasons – 'to be in charge of eating and activity habits' – is not a one-shot event but an ongoing process. So, in this way your reasons can help you keep things going and keep progress alive.

Keeping helpful plans going and maintaining a new weight can be a challenge

We have written a lot about some of the initial changes to eating and activity habits that will help with weight loss. However, for most people it is keeping habit changes going and maintaining weight loss that are the most challenging. Shifting attention to sustaining change and weight maintenance can be challenging and will require continued focus and effort.

Switching between being 'on' and 'off' a diet

People very often switch between being 'on a diet', where they are placing lots of attention and effort on what they do, to being 'off a diet', where they often try and avoid thinking about their eating and activity habits and usually abandon all previous changes. This is not a very helpful approach in the long term. However, if you follow the advice above, for example by making time to regularly review how things are going, paying attention gently and kindly to your progress, and developing plans for how to respond helpfully when things don't go to plan, you are more likely to feel in charge of your habits on a day-to-day basis.

Keep reviewing your list of reasons for managing your health and weight and think about adding more reasons – the reasons why it is important to keep these habit changes going. Think about all the benefits you have experienced as you've changed your habits and what you have learned in the process. For example, have you learned how to manage your physical hunger and food cravings in a different way? Have you managed social situations or other people's reactions better? Have you found a greater enjoyment in eating nourishing foods? Have you noticed how eating in this way affects how you feel and the energy you have? How being more active changes how you feel in your body and mind? Are you proud of keeping going even when things get tough?

Make sure you give yourself credit for all the effort and hard work you have put in and the things you have learned in the process. And when things are challenging be kind to yourself and ask for help and support if needed.

How and when to get professional help

At some point you may well think about getting some professional help. After all, this is what you might do with other health issues. In general, it's a good idea to consult a qualified professional. This section aims to let you know what your options are and to give you a realistic idea of what health professionals can – and can't – help with. We will deal with different types of help in turn.

Doctors

In general, there are two types of doctor you could see about weight and health, your family doctor or a specialist doctor, often an endocrinologist in a specialist weight-management clinic. Your family doctor is the most accessible and can help with a number of areas. They can work with you to explore some of the possible causes of weight gain, identify any associated medical conditions (or risks of) and develop a treatment plan for any conditions identified, such as raised blood pressure. Some family doctors may work with you to identify habit changes and provide ongoing support, or they may refer you to local programmes or other health professionals for additional support in managing weight.

In rare instances, there are specific medical conditions or prescribed medications that may be contributing to weight gain. The family doctor can discuss these with you, although in most instances this is not the explanation for weight gain.

The family doctor will always advise on food and activity changes as the foundation for improving health and managing weight. However, there are times when they may suggest using treatments in addition, but not instead of, these habit changes. These treatments include medications or surgery.

MEDICATION FOR MANAGING WEIGHT

Your family doctor may prescribe medication to help with weight management. However, at the time this book was published there were limited medications available for this purpose and what is available varies depending on the country you live in.

It's also possible to buy 'weight-loss' medication and supplements from commercial sources, for example over the internet. We will deal with these commercial drugs first.

There are a staggering number of different unregulated weight-loss pills and supplements on the market. There are three facts about nearly all of them you need to know:

1. There is little or no evidence they will help you lose weight.
2. They will cost you money.
3. There may be side effects associated with their use.

We would only advise using treatments that have evidence for their effectiveness and safety. This isn't the case for the majority of commercial pills and supplements. As such we would suggest saving your money, avoiding their use and focusing on approaches that are more likely to be helpful.

Prescription drugs available from your family doctor can be helpful for some people, although they work best when combined with changes to eating and activity habits. The medications available vary depending on your country of residence, but the options can be discussed with your family doctor. Some medications work by affecting the amount of fat your body absorbs from food, others work by reducing how hungry a person feels. As with all medications there are possible side effects and risks to their use that need careful discussion with your doctor.

Although medications can be very helpful for some people, it is important not to overestimate how much they can help in the long term. It is understandable to have high hopes for how drugs can help – a person might say, 'If I just get a bit of help from the drugs, I can change my habits.'

Of course, drugs may help and it's great when they do, but they work best when people also focus on making changes to eating and activity habits at the same time.

SURGERY

Surgery for weight loss (sometimes called bariatric surgery) is a very effective approach for managing severe and complex obesity, but it isn't suitable for everyone, and should never be undertaken without really thinking through possible long-term consequences. In many countries access to surgery requires referral to specialist clinics and a clear commitment to regular attendance at medical and nutrition appointments. These are part of the process of working out whether this is a treatment that may be helpful and which you're prepared to commit to for the rest of your life.

There are a variety of different surgical procedures available; some change the size or layout of the stomach, making it smaller, and others change the way food is processed. For the majority of people surgical treatment leads to quick and substantial weight loss in the first twelve to eighteen months, after which weight loss slows and eventually stops. Research has shown most people report big improvements to their quality of life as medical problems linked to their weight decrease, they take fewer medications, are able to move around more easily and generally feel better about themselves.

However, it is important to recognise there are side effects and risks with bariatric surgery. This isn't just the risk of the operation itself but also what might happen afterwards.

For surgical treatment to work well and to reduce certain side effects, such as vomiting after eating, it is important to change eating habits in the way the specialist clinics advise. There are also psychological consequences to surgery, for example if someone has become used to using food to cope with difficult emotions, this will not be an option after surgery. Therefore, it's important to consider what else will be put in place to help cope with difficulties.

It is also important to think through your expectations of surgery. Although it's a very effective treatment for those people who have severe and complex problems linked to their weight, it is not a quick, easy solution. It requires commitment to attend regular appointments, taking daily vitamin and mineral supplements, the same effort and dedication to change eating and activity habits as is needed with all other treatments, and a recognition that this does not come with a guarantee of being effective. There are a few people who really don't respond well to surgical treatment, either with poor weight loss or weight regain or who experience lots of complications after surgery. They are not the norm, but they do exist. People who lose very large amounts of weight may also be left with excess skin, which is not easily rectified and can be challenging to cope with emotionally.

However, despite these potential downsides surgery is a very effective and appropriate treatment for some people. If you are interested in exploring this further discuss it with your family doctor, who may then refer you to a specialist clinic.

Getting help with nutrition and dietary change

Changing eating habits is a central part of improving your health, caring for your body and managing weight, even if you add in drug or surgical treatment. There are many different people offering support and guidance on how best to do this and there isn't one approach that will suit everyone.

However, if you're seeking advice and support on nutrition it is important to ensure the professionals are properly qualified, otherwise you may be guided towards treatments with no evidence for their effectiveness or quality.

Dietitians are experts in food, nutrition and dietary change and importantly they are the only nutrition professionals regulated by law. In the UK, to use the title 'dietitian', they have to register with the Health and Care Professions Council (HCPC), have undertaken university training and follow a set of standards to protect the public and ensure the delivery of high-quality, evidence-based dietary treatment. Dietitians can assess and advise people on dietary treatments for general health improvement but also how to manage certain medical conditions such as diabetes or high blood pressure. To check if a dietitian is registered with the HCPC go to their website www.hcpc-uk.org and click on the *check the register* button. Dietitians work in the NHS and privately and some will specialise in weight management. To find a freelance dietitian check out www.freelancedietitians.org that searches by area and the type of advice you are seeking.

Unfortunately the term 'nutritionist' is not protected and

anyone can call themselves a nutritionist regardless of the level of training or competence to practise. To identify a good-quality nutritionist who has met high standards of nutrition education and provides evidence-based treatments it is helpful to check the UK Voluntary Registry of Nutritionists (UKVRN) run by the Association for Nutrition (AfN) www.associationfornutrition.org. Nutritionists provide advice on food and healthy eating but do not provide dietary treatment for medical conditions such as diabetes or high blood pressure.

Getting help for emotional problems

Emotional problems can be a serious block to managing weight. If you find yours are quite serious, it's a good idea to try to get some professional help.

There are two routes: first, to get help through your doctor, and second, to seek counselling or psychotherapy privately or from a voluntary organisation.

Your family doctor is your first point of contact for support with your emotional health. They can arrange two types of treatment for you: psychological therapy or medication. You might be offered medication first, because it is simpler, cheaper and can be started immediately.

Waiting lists for psychological therapy through the National Health Service can be long. However, there is much greater recognition of the value of psychological support and in response there have been some significant improvements. For example, in England all GPs can refer patients to the Improving Access to Psychological Therapy service (IAPT), and in some areas you will be able to contact this NHS service directly (search online for 'local IAPT'). If you are not in England, it is worth searching online for what other support is available locally, or contacting your health insurance company if you live outside the UK or have private health insurance.

If your doctor refers you for psychological help, this should be with a qualified practitioner. However, it's still helpful to have a look at the ideas for checking out your therapist that follow.

On the other hand, if you are offered medication, such as anti-depressants, there are a few things that it's useful to know.

Medication for emotional difficulties

Medication can be an incredibly useful treatment for emotional difficulties. However, many people do not like the idea of taking pills to help their mood. People often say pills 'don't really solve the problem'. This is partly true – and partly untrue. If the 'problem' is really long periods of sadness and crying, then pills sometimes will 'solve' it. However, it is more usual that pills give people the strength and energy *to solve their problems themselves*. It is hard to solve problems when you can hardly think because you're worrying all the time.

Medication can give you the freedom to help yourself.

People often have some other concerns about medication and can worry it's 'addictive' or it 'covers up the problem' but doesn't deal with it. Both of these are for the most part untrue. Modern forms of medication are usually not like the older drugs such as Valium (diazepam) that can cause dependence. They are usually made from a completely different type of chemical and do not cause people to become dependent in the same way. Even if your doctor does prescribe a Valium-type drug, you will not be given it for long enough to become dependent on it. When stopping any long-term medication, including antidepressants, it is important that you do this with the support of your doctor, as the medication you are on might need to be reduced gradually. As for 'covering up the problem', as we noted above, medication can give you enough clarity and stability to solve problems yourself. However, it cannot mend broken relationships or enable you to come to terms with really difficult life circumstances and you might want to seek additional support with this.

When taking medication, it is important to bear in mind that it doesn't work for everyone, and that sometimes it can have side effects. Sometimes there is a period when starting a new medication when you get side effects but do not feel any benefits. If this happens it is important to stick with the medication for a few weeks before deciding it's not working, but do consult your doctor or a pharmacist about any side effects you are concerned about.

The key to getting the most out of medication is to listen to your doctor, ask lots of questions and follow their advice, but also to remember the choice is yours about whether to take medication. Also, it's important to ask your doctor how long you should try a medication for before deciding if it's working for you or not. If you have been taking a medication as prescribed for several months and have not noticed any improvements, we would suggest you ask for a review. There might be another one that would work better for you, or other options.

Psychological support – psychotherapy and counselling

Alongside medication, or as an alternative, you might want to consider psychological help. As mentioned above, most therapists that you would be referred to by another health-care professional or insurance company are regulated and required to meet certain minimum professional standards. The most common type of therapists available through this route include clinical psychologists, counselling psychologists and counsellors.

Another option is to find a private therapist who you pay for yourself. Although we cannot give a complete guide here, we will cover three different topics: types of therapy, the qualifications of therapists and how to spot a reputable therapist.

There are lots of different types of therapy and counselling out there. We know some are helpful, because scientific studies have shown this. For example, CBT – cognitive-behavioural therapy – is a useful type of therapy for many (but certainly not all) people. The aim of many therapies is to help people find ways to respond to difficult life situations, thoughts, behaviours, moods and emotions, but not all therapists will also be able to provide the practical support needed to manage weight. Therefore you need to be clear about what you want and what you can realistically expect.

As CBT is one of the most evidence-based therapies available you might want to specifically look for a CBT therapist if you want weight-management support. This will either be a clinical psychologist whose training will have included CBT, or a therapist who has received additional training in CBT. The details of the main CBT regulating organisations in the UK and the USA are included in Appendix II.

Another consideration is the number of therapy sessions being offered. For CBT this can range from eight to twenty sessions, and your first session or second session with a therapist should include a clear conversation about the number of sessions and the reasons why the therapist is suggesting a certain number. Sometimes it is actually more helpful to just commit to fewer sessions and then check how things are going. Try a short-term therapy and then decide if you need or want extra sessions.

If a therapist strongly recommends you try long-term therapy without being able to give you reasons why, be cautious and ask them for more information.

We would suggest you only go to a therapist who is accredited by some kind of professional body and who receives regular supervision. The details of professional bodies such as the British Psychological Society are in Appendix II, which also provides more information on how to find a therapist and what to look for.

Finally, trust your feelings about your therapist. If you meet them for the first time and they seem competent, easy to talk to and open, this is a good sign. If it doesn't feel right, you may still decide to give it a go, but don't be afraid to 'shop around'. Below is a list of questions you can ask any therapist:

- What are your qualifications?
- Which professional body do you belong to?
- Which code of ethics do you follow?
- Do you have a qualified supervisor to discuss your work with?
- Is there a complaints procedure?
- For how many years have you been practising?
- How long is a session?
- How often are sessions held?
- What do you charge?
- Is there a cancellation fee?
- Is it a totally confidential service? (Be suspicious if they say 'yes' – would they really not tell anyone if you were obviously a risk to your own – or someone else's – health?)
- When might confidentiality be broken?
- How long might the therapy last for?
- How does therapy end?

These questions were put together by POPAN – the Prevention of Professional Abuse Network (*details in Appendix II*) – though the note in brackets is our own. POPAN also has some good advice on warning signs that things might not be going well with your therapist – have a look at their website or phone them if you are concerned.

Some parting words

This is the end of the book.

We wish you every success in managing your health and weight. Remember, the helpful approach is to explore and really understand your habits – why you behave in the way you do with eating and activity – and then to experiment with changes until you find an approach that works for you. This takes time and patience and often many attempts before you hit on changes that are helpful. It's important to be kind to yourself during the process.

Don't underestimate yourself, no matter how many times you have tried to make changes to your habits. Making assumptions about what you can and cannot do isn't helpful and can stop you from even trying – remember, these are just thoughts! Each time you try to change, you have more experience than previously, and this can be brought to your new attempt.

We hope you find the ideas and tools presented in this book helpful and can use them to build up your knowledge and skills to make long-term changes to improve your health and happiness.   **Best of luck!**

Appendix I

Planning and recording

Body mass index

	5'0"	5'1"	5'2"	5'3"	5'4"	5'5"	5'6"	5'7"	5'8"	5'9"	5'10"	5'11"	6'0"	6'1"	6'2"	6'3"	6'4"
9st	25	24	23	22	22	21	20	20	19	19	18	18	17	17	16	16	15
9.5st	26	25	24	24	23	22	21	21	20	20	19	19	18	18	17	17	16
10st	27	26	26	25	24	23	23	22	21	21	20	20	19	18	18	17	17
10.5st	29	28	27	26	25	24	24	23	22	22	21	21	20	19	19	18	18
11st	30	29	28	27	26	26	25	24	23	23	22	21	21	20	20	19	19
11.5st	31	30	29	29	28	27	26	25	24	24	23	22	22	21	20	20	20
12st	33	32	31	30	29	28	27	26	26	25	24	23	23	22	22	21	20
12.5st	34	33	32	31	30	29	28	27	27	26	25	24	24	23	22	22	21
13st	36	34	33	32	31	30	29	29	28	27	26	25	25	24	23	23	22
13.5st	37	36	35	33	32	31	31	30	29	28	27	26	26	25	24	24	23
14st	38	37	36	35	34	33	32	31	30	29	28	27	27	26	25	24	24
14.5st	40	38	37	36	35	34	33	32	31	30	29	28	28	27	26	25	25
15st	41	40	38	37	36	35	34	33	32	31	30	29	28	28	27	26	26
15.5st	42	41	40	38	37	36	35	34	33	32	31	30	29	29	28	27	26
16st	44	42	41	40	38	37	36	35	34	33	32	31	30	30	29	28	27
16.5st	45	44	42	41	40	38	37	36	35	34	33	32	31	30	30	29	28
17st	46	45	43	42	41	40	38	37	36	35	34	33	32	31	31	30	29
17.5st	48	46	44	43	42	41	40	38	37	36	35	34	33	32	31	31	30
18st	49	48	46	45	44	42	41	39	38	37	36	35	34	33	32	31	31
18.5st	51	49	47	46	44	43	42	41	39	38	37	36	35	34	33	32	32
19st	52	50	49	47	46	44	43	42	40	39	38	37	36	35	34	33	32
19.5st	53	52	50	48	47	45	44	43	42	40	39	38	37	36	35	34	33
20st	55	53	51	50	48	47	45	44	43	41	40	39	38	36	36	35	34
20.5st	56	54	52	51	49	48	46	45	44	42	41	40	39	37	37	36	35
21st	57	56	54	52	50	49	47	46	45	43	42	41	40	38	38	37	36
21.5st	59	57	55	53	52	50	49	47	46	44	43	42	41	39	39	38	37
22st	60	58	56	55	53	51	50	48	47	45	44	43	42	41	40	38	37

Calculate your BMI by finding your weight (in stone) on the left and then your height (in feet and inches) above. The number that you read off from the table is your BMI.

Questioning and expanding your thinking

Summary of the process

You will need a pen and paper. Here's the whole process. It is not complicated – it boils down to working out what's bothering you, and then checking out your view of the situation. Remember to refer back to chapter 2 to remind yourself about the full details of this process.

1. Pinpoint the thought.
   Explain the thought fully.
   Summarise the most upsetting or difficult part.
2. Question it.
   Use the questions below.
3. Expand your thinking.
   Find three alternative views of the situation.

Long list of questions

Below is a list of ten questions that can usefully be applied to almost any thought. Use this 'long' list when you are starting to use this process. It is also useful for very difficult or 'stuck' thoughts. Of course, not all questions will apply to the particular thought you are dealing with.

1. What is the evidence for this thought? What is the evidence against it?
2. What are other ways of thinking about this situation?
3. How would another person see this situation? What would I say to my best friend or someone I loved if they were in the same situation?

4. What are the advantages and disadvantages of thinking this way?

5. When I am not feeling this way, do I think about this type of situation differently? How?

6. Am I asking questions that have no answers?

7. Five years from now, if I look back at this situation, will I look at it any differently? Will I pay attention to other parts of the situation that I'm ignoring now?

8. Are there any small things that show my thoughts aren't true? Am I ignoring them or not taking them seriously?

9. Am I blaming myself for something over which I do not have complete control? Am I forgetting that other people are responsible for their own behaviour (and I'm not responsible for what they do)?

10. Am I always thinking that things will go badly? Am I exaggerating how bad things would be if they did go wrong?

Short list of questions

When you have had some practice in questioning and expanding thoughts with the long list, you may find you just need to use the questions below. If you find a particularly difficult thought, then go back to the long list.

- Is this thought true (and unbiased)?
- Is this thought helpful?
- What are other ways of looking at the situation?

PHYSICAL ACTIVITY RECORD FORM

Time	Moods or sensations	Activity	Time (minutes) L M V★
06.00			
07.00			
08.00			
09.00			
10.00			
11.00			
12.00			
13.00			
14.00			
15.00			
16.00			

17.00			
18.00			
19.00			
20.00			
21.00			
22.00			
23.00			
24.00			
01.00			

* Use this column to record the intensity of your activity. Remember, any movement counts, and aim for moderate level when you can.

Light = gentle activity, general moving around

Moderate = talk but can't sing, a little bit warmer, slightly raised heart rate

Vigorous = out of breath, sweating, heart beating fast

Important automatic thoughts:
(Remember to use the
steps discussed previously to
investigate these)

Number of minutes being
active:

Number of steps:

EATING RECORD FORM

Situation and Time	Moods or sensations	What you ate

Important automatic thoughts:

PLANNING FORMS

ACTIVITY/EXERCISE PLANS

- What exactly is the plan? (Amounts Count!)
- What help do you need for your plan? Whose support would be helpful?
- When are you going to start, and when are you going to check and review your plan?

EATING/FOOD PLANS

- What exactly is the plan? (Amounts Count!)
- What help do you need for your plan? Whose support would be helpful?
- When are you going to start, and when are you going to check and review your plan?

REASONS

- What are the good reasons for spending time and effort making these plans work?

Problem-solving

Problem-solving is a critical part of managing weight long-term. Practise these techniques and use them a lot! Remember that actually going through the steps with pen and paper is the only way to do it. If you try to 'just think the problem through', you may be successful, but you will more often be disappointed. Use the technique fully.

A quick summary of the process

These are the basic steps of problem-solving:

1. Define your problem.
2. Make up lots of alternative solutions.
3. Analyse your alternatives.
4. Try out your solution(s).
5. See how it went – and do it again!

Below are some helpful tips for each stage of the process:

DEFINE YOUR PROBLEM

- What exactly is the problem? Try to be really clear.
- Are you sure this is your problem? Check you are working on the right issue.
- Are you trying to solve a huge problem? Try to break it down into smaller ones and work on one of these.

MAKE UP LOTS OF ALTERNATIVE SOLUTIONS

- Remember that anything goes. Do not criticise or reject any ideas at this stage.
- Start off with some silly ideas if you get stuck. They help to get things going.
- Keep going until you have plenty of alternatives. Make sure you have at least five, preferably ten!

ANALYSE YOUR ALTERNATIVES

- Throw out the options that really will not work.
- Work out how good the other options would be in the short, medium and long term.
- Always remember you are trying to build positive habits that will stay with you.

TRY OUT YOUR SOLUTION(S)

- Make your solution a SMART solution (*see chapter 6*).
- Make sure you really try your solution out in real life. This is where you will learn most.

SEE HOW IT WENT - AND DO IT AGAIN!

- Be honest about how well it worked.
- Do not be critical if your solution only produced a small change. A small genuine change is better than a big change that will not last.
- If your solution did not work, this is not a 'failure'. Instead it means that you have just learned something important. Learning what does not work is central to the process.
- Problem-solving is a repeated process of being flexible and creative. Keep going and try it again!

Keeping track with a smartphone

We recommend using your smartphone to help you keep track, including using its pedometer or step-counter app to monitor physical activity, particularly if you don't feel like paying for a separate device like a Fitbit. Beyond this, there are many other apps that might be useful and really can help you change your habits. Although it's not possible to suggest any specific apps here as there is such a huge range and these change very quickly, we would suggest searching online for reviews of the type of apps you might find helpful: habit tracking, physical activity, healthy eating or relaxation are helpful searches to start with. There are various food-diary apps that can help with monitoring eating – they make recording 'on the go' relatively easy. However, do be careful about apps that stipulate very rigid or restrictive dieting approaches as these may cause more problems than they solve.

When you start using an app, it's worth checking in with yourself about any thoughts or feelings that come up and, using your CBT skills, asking yourself: 'Does this app help me to understand myself better, and to change my habits for the long term?' When you are setting goals and looking to change what you do, apps from the 'habit' family can be very useful. These usually allow you to define goals in SMART terms, and you can often set them to 'prompt' so you keep on track. They often provide a graph of your progress and this can be helpful in visualising how things are going. Many habit-tracking apps don't focus specifically on weight, but if you do decide to use a weight-focused one we would encourage you to choose an app that includes behaviour change, CBT and relaxation/mindfulness strategies. For example, some food-diary apps allow you to track foods or situations that trigger episodes of unplanned overeating.

It's helpful to recognise that different apps work for different people. For example, 'calorie counter' apps might help some people to be more aware of portion sizes and recognise in a helpful way areas where they can focus changes. ('Amounts Count' – chapter 3.) However, for other people, who may have yo-yo dieted and 'counted calories' for decades, these apps might not be helpful and may divert attention away from where they really need to focus change, like the need to deal with other people differently (chapter 8). Similarly, 'weight tracker' apps can be really helpful for some people and not others. So, another good question is: 'Does this app help me to focus on issues that will help me in the long term?' Good luck with choosing.

Appendix II

Taking it further

Useful organisations

Professional UK organisations

These organisations represent particular professions. They usually hold information about their own profession and have lists of registered professionals/therapists.

British Dietetic Association (BDA)
This is the professional organisation for dietitians.
Tel: 0121 200 8080
www.bda.uk.com
email: info@bda.uk.com

To find a freelance dietitian, check out www.freelance dietitians.org. This website has a search function that allows you to look for freelance and private-practice dietitians by location and specialist clinical area.

Association of Nutrition
Professional organisation for registered nutritionists that holds the UK voluntary register of nutritionists (UKVRN). This is the only register of nutritionists recognised by the NHS and Public Health England and identifies nutritionists who have met high educational standards and practice in line with scientific evidence.
www.associationfornutrition.org

Health & Care Professions Council
This organisation regulates health, psychological and social-work professionals. Dietitians and psychologists must be registered with this organisation and it is possible to search the register to check if your health professional is currently registered. They also set the standards for training and education and take action if professionals do not meet the expected standards.
Tel: 0300 500 6184
www.hcpc-uk.org

The British Psychological Society (BPS)
Professional organisation for psychologists, including clinical psychologists, counselling psychologists and health psychologists.
Tel: 0116 254 9568
www.bps.org.uk
email: enquiries@bps.org.uk

US organisations

Academy of Nutrition & Dietetics
As well as being a site providing useful resources on eating well, it also holds the national database of registered dietitians/nutritionists and can be searched by location or area of expertise.
www.eatright.org
www.eatright.org/find-an-expert

Association for Behavioral and Cognitive Therapies (ABCT, formerly AABT)
Clinical directory and referral service.
Tel: (00 1) 212 647 1890
www.abct.org

National Institute of Mental Health (NIMH)
Working to improve mental health.
Tel: (00 1) 301 443 4513
www.nimh.nih.gov
email: nimhinfo@nih.gov

Therapy

These organisations represent people practising a particular type of psychological therapy. They ensure a certain level of training and a code of conduct. However, the people involved may not have had the same comprehensive training as a healthcare professional. The exception is the BABCP (immediately below), which does require professional qualification in a 'core profession' (e.g. psychology, nursing, social work) to be accredited as a CBT therapist.

British Association for Behavioural & Cognitive Psychotherapies (BABCP)
Professional organisation for CBT therapists in the UK and Ireland. Provides information and a list of trained therapists.
Tel: 0161 797 4484
www.babcp.com
email: babcp@babcp.com

British Association for Counselling and Psychotherapy (BACP)
Lists of UK counsellors and psychotherapists.
Tel: 01455 883316
www.bacp.co.uk
email: bacp@bacp.co.uk

British Psychoanalytic Council (BPC)
Organisation for people practising more long-term psycho-therapy/psychoanalytical treatments.
Tel: 020 7561 9240
www.bpc.org.uk
email: mail@bpc.org.uk

UK Council for Psychotherapy (UKCP)
Information about psychotherapy. Holds its own register of psychotherapists.
Tel: 020 7014 9955
www.psychotherapy.org.uk
email: info@psychotherapy.org.uk

Experts by experience

The National Weight Control Registry
Details all the evidence from the NWCR we mention throughout the book. You can also join the NWCR through this link.
www.nwcr.ws

Voluntary/self-help

BEAT
Charity providing information and support for people affected by bulimia, anorexia, binge eating.
Tel: 0808 801 0677
www.beateatingdisorders.co.uk
email: help@ beateatingdisorders.co.uk

MIND
Information, support and other resources on mental health.
Tel: 0300 123 3393
www.mind.org.uk
email: info@mind.org.uk

Self-Compassion
A great website developed by Dr Kristin Neff drawing together years of research on being kind to ourselves. Includes practical exercises and audio-guided meditations.
self-compassion.org

Weight Concern
Provides information and written resources around being overweight and obesity.
www.weightconcern.com
email: enquiries@weightconcern.org.uk

Are services for overweight people in your area inadequate?

Services across the UK are can vary a great deal. If you feel that weight-management services in your area are inadequate you can contact your MP and let them know how you feel. You can find out your MP's details at: www. parliament.cuk/mps-lords-and-offices/mps

Useful websites

These websites contain useful information about managing weight and its health consequences.

www.bdaweightwise.com
Very useful website from the British Dietetic Association that provides some practical advice on changing eating habits.

www.wlsinfo.org.uk
Weight Loss Surgery Info. This website provides comprehensive support, information and guidance for people thinking about or who have already had bariatric surgery.

www.nhs.uk
NHS website providing comprehensive information about NHS services and self-help information on common conditions. Includes 'Live Well' section on dietary and physical activity advice, e.g. structured 'couch to 5k' programme for people new to jogging, using podcasts and videos.

www.nutrition.org.uk
British Nutrition Foundation. Aims to provide scientifically sound information about nutrition.

www.weightconcern.com
Weight Concern charity, as listed under 'Organisations' on page 380. Contains good material on weight, health risks and nutrition and activity.

For professionals and campaigners

www.aso.org.uk
The Association for the Study of Obesity. Mainly for researchers and professionals. Contains a useful 'information centre' with fact sheets.

www.bda.uk.com/regionsgroups/groups/obesity
BDA Obesity specialist group. For dietitians working in Obesity Management in the UK. Evidence summaries, training events, news and resources provided for dietitians working in this area.

www.obesity.org
Obesity Society. American scientific–membership campaign group.

www.uconnruddcenter.org/weight-bias-stigma
The Rudd Center for Food Policy & Obesity.
A US non-profit, university-run research and public policy

organisation promoting solutions to childhood obesity, poor diet and weight bias through research and policy.

https://www.scope-elearning.org/Saba/Web_wdk/EU2PRD0110/index/prelogin.rdf
SCOPE – strategic centre for Obesity Professional Education. Provides an internationally recognised certification in obesity management delivered via online educational modules.

Useful reading

Binge-eating and bulimia

Fairburn, Christopher, *Overcoming Binge Eating*, New York: Guilford Press, 2013
Very clear and practical.

Goss, Kenneth, *The Compassionate Mind Approach to Beating Overeating*, London: Robinson, 2011
Helps readers to understand and work with strong food cravings and attachments whilst paying attention to biological and emotional needs.

Schmidt, Ulrike, Treasure, Janet and Alexander, June, *Getting Better Bit(e) by Bit(e): A Survival Kit for Sufferers of Bulimia Nervosa and Binge Eating Disorders*, Hove, UK: Psychology Press, 2015
Good, wide-ranging book including chapters on being assertive and dealing with a history of abuse.

Cognitive behavioural therapy

Burns, David D., *Feeling Good: The New Mood Therapy*, New York: Avon Books, 2000
Large book containing a wide range of material, from managing depression to relationships.

Greenberger, Dennis and Padesky, Christine, *Mind over Mood: Change How You Feel by Changing the Way You Think*, New York: Guilford Press, 2015
Practical, lots of monitoring sheets, examples, handouts, etc; very good for developing CBT skills.

Depression and general low self-regard

Fennell, Melanie, *Overcoming Low Self-Esteem*, London: Robinson, 2016
Strongly recommended for those whose poor self-esteem is a long-standing problem.

Gilbert, Paul, *Overcoming Depression*, London: Robinson, 2009
Excellent – detailed, practical, with case studies.

Relationship difficulties and communication skills

Christensen, Andrew, Doss, Brian. D. and Jacobson, Neil S., *Reconcilable Differences: Rebuild Your Relationship by Rediscovering the Partner You Love – Without Losing Yourself*, New York: Guilford Press, 2014
Highly recommended for clear communication strategies, based on research.

Quilliam, Susan, *Stop Arguing, Start Talking: The 10-Point Plan for Couples in Conflict*, London: Vermillion, 2001
Practical, readable and sometimes humorous book.

Rosenberg, Marshall, *Nonviolent Communication: A Language of Life: Life-Changing Tools for Healthy Relationships*. Encinitas: Puddle Dancer Press, 2015
An international bestseller. Helps to identify and express needs in a wide range of relationships and friendships, including with a partner, as well as at work and in day-to-day life.

Index

Note: page numbers in **bold** refer to diagrams.

abuse 8, 9, 319–22, 357
achievements, recognition 231–2
aerobic activity 156–7
alcohol intake 105, 205–6
'all or nothing' thinking 64
anger 32, 266, 325, 326
anorexia nervosa 9, 23
anxiety 249, 266
appointments 331–2
apps 332, 372–4
  'habit' 224, 228, 372–3
Association for Nutrition (AfN)
  351, 376
Atkins diet 181, 182, 190–1
automatic thoughts 59–77, **366,
  367**
  'appearance' 66–71
  becoming aware of your 66–77,
    84–5
  biased 63–4, 85–7
  dealing with 77–90
  and emotions 63–5, 71–3, 74–8,
    84, 89–90
  examples of 67–71
  and expanding your thinking
    77–8, 83–4, 362–3
  limited perspective of 65
  negative 62–4, 66–71, 78,
    84

pinpointing your most import-
    ant 73–7, 88–9
  positive 66
  questioning your 77–83, 84,
    88–90
  recording your **108**, 109, **112**
  unhelpful nature of 65
  untrue 63–4
  about weight loss 67
  where to 'find' 71

babies 253
'bad' foods 168–9, 172–3
bariatric surgery 348–9, 381
beans 194, 195
behaviour 21
  changing patterns of 21
  recording 98, 99, 104, 108,
    113–14, 116–17, 120
  and setbacks 336
beliefs 58–90
'Big Things' 120, 121, 122
binge-eating disorder 23
binging 14, 23, 170–1, **171**, 383
blaming others 302
  see also self-blame
blood pressure 52
  high 26, 130, 346, 350, 351
blood-sugar levels 172, 187, 342

bodies
  body ideals 7–9
  body shape 134–5
  feelings/attitudes towards our
    7–9
body mass index (BMI) 23, 25–6,
  361
boredom 146, 266
brain 198
breakfasts, habits 18–19, 255–6,
  259
breathing techniques 276
British Heart Foundation 200,
  201, 204
British Medical Journal 9
British Psychological Society 355,
  377
'Broken Plans' 120, 121, 122
'broken record' technique
  314–16
budgeting 93–4
bulimia 23, 383

cabbage soup diet 181, 183
calories
  requirements 175–6
  underestimating intake 6
Cambridge diet 180
cancer 130, 192, 193, 199, 203
carbohydrates, refined 198–9, 200
case studies
  Dave 269–70
  Jackie 47–9, 178–9, 252–4, 285,
    342–3
  Kirsty 96–100, 105–12, **106–8**,
    111–12, 154, 229–30,
    236–42, 298–9, 305–6,
    313–16
  Linda 138, 197–8
  Lisa 131
  Patricia 263–4, 265
  Pauline 255–6
  Pete 59–60, 62–3, 79–83, 262,

    298–9, 304–7, 309–10, 312,
    335
  Sandra 170–1, 175–7, 179–83,
    321–6, 332
catastrophizing (thought error) 64
CBT *see* cognitive behavioural
  therapy
cereals 198
  see also whole grains
changes, making 125–357
  in daily life 212–46
  and dealing with other people's
    reactions 283–327
  and emotional eating 247–82
  from the inside out 92–3
  keeping it going 328–57
  see also eating habits, changing;
    motivation to change; physi-
    cal activity habits, changing
children, and parental weight gain
  15, 60, 253
cognitive behavioural therapy
  (CBT) 20, 58–9, 234, 334,
  336, 339–40, 354–5, 373, 384
comfort eating 9, 247–8, 252–4
commercial weight-management
  groups 187–8
communication skills 385
  see also other people's reactions,
    dealing with
computers 150–1
confidence
  and physical activity 143–4
  and weight loss 16, 18
cool downs 156
Cooper, Peter 23
coping approaches 324, 334–5
cortisol levels 258
counselling 351, 354–7
crisps 5

daily life, making changes in
  212–46

and bad ideas 222–3
and planning 213–21, 223–33, 242
and problem-solving 233–43
and progress checking 229–33
and temptations 222–3
and weight loss 243–6
daily routines 156–7, 165, 215–16
debt problems 11
dehydration 105, 167
depression 130, 249, 384
  post-natal 253
detoxification 184
diabetes 36–7, 47–8, 130, 187, 193, 342, 350–1
  see also prediabetes
diazepam (Valium) 353
dieticians 350
diets 1–3, 162
  Atkins diet 181, 182, 190–1
  cabbage soup diet 181, 183
  Cambridge diet 180
  fad-type 165, 184–5
  food elimination diets 11
  learning from past dieting experience 179–84
  liquid formula diets 189–90
  low-carbohydrate diets 190–1
  low-fat diets 186
  meal replacement diets 188–9
  Mediterranean diet 191–2
  'Perfect Diet' 14–16
  popular 184–92
  professional help with 350–1
  quick fix diets 10–13
  safe and healthy diets 185–9
  switching between being 'on' and 'off' 344–5
  thinking you can find the right one 163–5
  unhelpful beliefs about 163–6
  Weight Watchers 180, 182
  yo-yo dieting 2, 3, 222–3

difficulties, overcoming 37–43
digital technology 224, 228, 332, 372–4
discrimination, against large-sized people 8, 9, 50–2, 284, 319–22
distractions 270–2
doctors 345–9, 351–4

eat well principles 192–207
  alcohol 205–6
  fish 201
  fruit 192–8, **193**
  healthy fats 201–4
  lean meats 201
  portion sizes 204
  pulses 201
  soft drinks 206–7
  vegetables 192–8, **193**
  whole grains 198–200
eating
  beliefs about 'normal' levels of 295, 297–9, 301
  comfort eating 9, 247–8, 252–4
  irregular 255–7, 259
  recording your patterns of 104–5, 110–14, **110–12**, 116–18, 122
  see also emotional eating; overeating
eating disorders 9, 23, 383
eating habits, changing 17, 22, 24–5, 162–211, 214–17, 240–1, 244, 246, 253, 278
  and bariatric surgery 349
  and the eat well principles 192–207
  and food labels 207–10, **208**
  helpful approaches to 179–84
  and helpful beliefs 172–3
  and keeping it going 328–30, 343, 344
  and medication 347–8

other people's influence on
   283–4, 286–90
and popular diets 184–92
professional help with 350–1
reinforcement 277
and unhelpful beliefs 163–72
and weight control 173–9
eating plans 162–3, 223–4, 226,
   269
and other people 284–5, 287–9,
   291, 293–5, 300
Eating Record Form 257,
   367–8
emotional difficulties, getting
   help with 278, 351–7,
   377–9
emotional eating 247–82
   and acting on feelings 262–4
   and back-up plans 278–81
   and different emotions 249–50
   and distractions 270–2
   and emotional acceptance
      267–8
   and emotional aftershocks
      259–60
   and getting familiar with your
      feelings 260–2
   and holding steady 277–80
   and motivations for change
      268–9
   and pressing pause 275–7
   and recognising emotions 251–5
   replacements for 269–70
   and self-talk 272–4
   and sensations 249–50
   starting work with 255–60
   and thoughts 265–7
   and the transient nature of
      emotions 264–5
emotional hunger 102–4
   see also food cravings
emotions
   acceptance 267–8

and automatic thinking 63–5,
   71–3, 74–8, 84, 89–90
coping with 25
positive 102
recognition 251–5
recording 100
regarding weight loss 32
transient nature of 264–5
see also feelings; specific emotions
endocrinologists 345
endosperm 198
energy balance 173–5, **174**
energy burning 108
environments 286–90

Facebook 8
facts, checking your 301–2, 338
Fairburn, Christopher 23
family doctors 345–6, 347, 351–2
fast food 6
fat metabolisers 189
fat-free foods 169–70, 208
fatigue/tiredness 105, 164,
   258–9, 266
fats
   healthy 201–4
   hidden 170
   saturated 202
   unsaturated 202
   see also high-fat foods; low-fat
      foods
fear 250
'feel-good' factor 129, 134, 135
feelings 21–2
   and automatic thinking 71–3,
      74–8, 84, 89–90
   coping with 25
   and emotional hunger 102
   following your 72–3, 74–5, 84
   mixed 302
   willingness to tolerate unpleas-
      ant 326–7
   see also emotions; sensations

fibre 199
fish 201
Fitbits 372
'Five Years' exercise 43–50
fizzy drinks 105, 206–7
food
  'bad' 168–9, 172–3
  changes 162–3
  eating your children's 15, 60
  fast 6
  fat-free 169–70, 208
  fried 6
  'good' 168–9, 172–3
  high-energy 7
  high-fat 203, 208, 209
  high-fibre 199
  'labelling' 168–9, 172–3
  low-fat 203, 207, 208, 209
  low-sugar 169–70
  as punishment 248
  reduced-fat 208, 209
  as reward 136, 138, 248, 277
  starchy **193**, 194, 195
food cravings 136, 164, 247, 277
  and distractions 270–2
  and thoughts 266
  understanding the emotional
    nature of 102–4
  and watching TV 151
food elimination diets 11
food intake
  awareness of your levels of 94–5
  recording 95–9, 98–9, 113
  reduction 3
food labels 170, 204, 207–10,
  208
food tastes/preferences 165
forgetfulness 115
framing, positive 42–3, 54
Freeman, Christopher 23
fried food 6
fruit 192–8, **193**
fruit juices 195

fullness levels, recording **103**,
  104, **110–11**
fun, having 231
future, envisioning the 43–50

general practitioners (GPs) 345–6,
  347, 351–2
germ 198
goals
  SMART 373
  weight 338–41, 343
'good' foods 168–9, 172–3
Graham, Patricia 23
grounding technique, 5-4-3-2-1
  275–7
guilt 54, 116, 256, 262, 318–19

habits
  changing 18–21, 212–17, 219,
    221, 223, 227, 232–3, 249,
    342–3, 357
  formation 216
  getting used to new 219
  'habit' apps 224, 228, 372–3
  and mental health 249
  recording 96–9
  understanding your day-to-day
    93–5
  see also eating habits, changing;
    physical activity habits,
    changing
happiness 16, 18
HbA1c measure 342
HCPC see Health and Care
  Professions Council
head hunger see emotional hunger
health
  improvement 22
  and physical activity 139
  and weight gain 50–2
Health and Care Professions
  Council (HCPC) 350, 377
health conditions 130, 148–9, 165

see also mental health problems; *specific conditions*

health risks 36–7

heart disease 26, 130, 187, 192, 193, 199, 203

help
  asking for 310–13
  professional 345–57

high blood pressure 26, 130, 346, 350, 351

high-energy foods, natural human preference for 7

high-fat foods 203, 208, 209

high-fibre foods 199

hunger
  and alcohol intake 205
  awareness of the different types of 100–4
  emotional 102–4
  and meal-skipping 170, 171
  physical 101, 102–4, 135–6, 255–8
  recording 100–4, **110–11**, 122
  and thoughts 265

hunger scale 103, **103**

ideal (goal) weight 338–41, 343

Improving Access to Psychological Therapy (IAPT) 352

Instagram 8

insulin sensitivity 258

job stress 112

jogging 149

Johnson, Michael 339

keeping it going 328–57
  getting professional help 345–57
  getting stuck and going backwards 333–8
  knowing where to stop 338–45

and slipping backwards 328, 329–32

switching between being 'on' and 'off' a diet 344–5

'labelling' foods 168–9, 172–3

laxatives 23

lifestyle activities 151–3

liquid formula diets 189–90

listening skills 310–13

living for the moment 50–3

loneliness 164

low glycaemic index (low-GI) diets 187

low-carbohydrate diets 190–1

low-fat foods 203, 207, 208, 209

low-sugar foods 169–70

meal replacement diets 188–9

meal-skipping 170–2, **171**, 255–6, 259

meats, lean 201

media representation 8–9

medication
  for emotional problems 351, 352–3
  for weight management 346–8

Mediterranean diet 191–2

mental health problems 249

metabolic rate 177–8

models 8–9

moods, recording 98–101, **106–7**, 108, **110–11**, 112, 120–1

motivation to change 17, 24, 31–57, 341–3
  defining motivation 33–6
  and emotional eating 268–9
  and the 'Five Years' exercise 43–50
  and guilt 54
  personal reasons behind 33, 35, 55–6
  and positive framing 42–3, 54

pulling it all together 54–6
and starting plans 225, 226
things that reduce 50–3, 56
weight loss motivations 17, 24,
    31–57, 341–3
multipacks 5
muscle mass, and weight loss 130,
    176, 177
music 271

National Health Service (NHS)
    350, 351–2, 381
National Weight Control
    Registry (NWCR) 16–18,
    19, 224, 339–40, 379
needs, communicating your
    302–3
Neff, Dr Kristin 274
negative automatic thoughts
    62–4, 66–71, 78, 84
negotiation 303–19
norms 295–9, 301
nurses 47–8
nutrition, professional help with
    350–1, 382
nutritionists 350–1

other people's judgements,
    regarding your weight 50–2
other people's reactions, dealing
    with 283–327
and asking for help 310–13
checking your view of the
    problem 300–3
and encouragement/discourage-
    ment 292–4, 301–2
and feeling guilty 318–19
and feeling selfish 318–19
and how other people treat you
    284, 292–300
and influences on your plans
    284–92
and lack of support 290–5

and listening to others 310–13
and making your own plan
    319–27
and norms 295–9, 301
and other people's choices
    284–90
and picking your moment
    307–8
and positive influencers 284
and raising issues and negotiat-
    ing 303–19
regarding your weight 8, 9,
    50–2, 284, 319–22
and saboteurs 14, 25, 292–3,
    304–19
and talking clearly and forcefully
    313–19
and 'talking from above' 308–10
and telling people what you
    want/need 302–3
and willingness to put up with
    unpleasant feelings 326–7
and your environment 286–90
overeating 4–6, 7, 256
as act of rebellion 9
alternatives to 271–2
and comfort eating 9, 247–8,
    252–4
and discrimination against
    overweight 9
and distractions 270–2
emotional 102–3, 248–50, 252,
    254–5, 257–9, 263, 268,
    269, 272–4, 277–81
reactions to 116–17
recording 122
replacements for 269–70
and sleep levels 258–9
and 'surfing the urge' 271–2
overweight
causes of 4–9
discrimination against 8, 9, 284,
    319–22

feelings/attitudes towards 8
global prevalence 1
working out your levels of 25–7
overweight services, national
    variations in 381

'Parkrun' 149
pedometers 109, 141, 154–5, 372
'permission-giving' thoughts 112
perspective-taking 322–5
physical activity 3
  aerobic activity 156–7
  as alternative to overeating 271
  beliefs about 'normal' levels of
      295–7, 299, 301
  and quick fix diets 12
  recording 95–9, 104–9, **106–7**,
      113–14, 118, 122, 141–2
  strength training 140
  and weight loss 176
physical activity habits, chang-
      ing 17, 22, 24–5, 127–61,
      214–17, 244
  amounts of 139–41
  awareness of your levels of 94,
      95, 141–2
  barriers to 142–50
  benefits of 129–32, 134–5,
      140–1, 145–6
  and boredom 146
  and calorie-burning 137–8
  disappointment with the results
      of 148
  enjoyment 131
  expense of 145–6
  falling levels of 7
  and fear of injury 148–9
  and 'feeling the burn' 133
  finding time for 131, 144–5
  helpful activities 150–7
  hoping for too much too soon
      134–5
  how it applies to you 157–9

and hunger 135–7
keeping it going 328–30, 343,
    344
knowing what not to do 132–8
knowing what to do 139–42
lack of confidence with 143–4
lack of motivation for 147–8
and medication 347–8
moderate 139–40
negative experiences of 127,
    132, 142
not feeling like it 146–8
other people's influence on 284,
    287–90
personal meanings of 128
role in keeping weight off
    131–2
routines 156–7
safety concerns 149
too much, too soon 132–3
vigorous 139, 140
and worries about your appear-
    ance 150
physical activity plans 223–4, 226,
    269
  and other people 284–5, 287–9,
      291, 293–5, 300
physical activity record form
    364–6
physical reactions 21
planning 213–21, 223–33, 242,
    359–74
  back-up plans 278–81
  'Broken Plans' 120, 121, 122
  and emotional eating 278–81
  learning from 232–3
  making successful plans 213–16
  and other people 284–92,
      319–27
  putting plans into action 227–8
  SMART planning 216–21,
      223–4, 227, 242, 247
  starting to plan 223–7

timescales 219–20
see also eating plans; physical
    activity plans
pleasure 266
POPAN *see* Prevention of
    Professional Abuse Network
portion sizes 204
    cutting down on 220
    fish 201
    fruit 194–5
    portion distortion 4–6, 204
    recording 104–5
    vegetables 194–5
positive emotions 102
positive framing 42–3, 54
positive thinking 58, 66
post-natal depression 253
prediabetes 175
'pressing pause' 275–7
Prevention of Professional Abuse
    Network (POPAN) 357
problem-solving 233–43, 320–2,
    337, 369–71
    alternative solutions 237–9, 371
    analysing alternatives 240–2,
        371
    defining the problem 236–7,
        370
    evaluation 242–3, 372
    trying out your solution 242,
        371
professional help 345–57
progress checking 229–33, 341–3
pseudo-cereals 198
psychotherapy 351, 354–7
pulses 194, 195, 201
punishments, food as 248

quality of life 22
quick fix diets
    fad theories 12–13
    long-term failure 10–13
    and missing out exercise 12

restrictive/boring nature of
    10–11
short-termism of 11–12

realism 218–19, 339–41
recording information 95–123,
    359–74
    'Big Things' 120, 121, 122
    'Broken Plans' 120, 121, 122
    common problems 114–19
    duration 114
    general principles of 100–5
    how to 113–14
    keeping private 119
    making sense of it all 120–2
    Overall Amounts 121, 122
    useful information 122–3
reduced-fat foods 208, 209
regret 102, 116–17
relationship difficulties 385
responsibilities 165
restaurants 6
rewards 232
    food as 136, 138, 248, 277
routines 156–7, 165, 215–16
running coaches 119

saboteurs, weight loss 14, 25,
    292–3, 304–19
sadness 265, 268, 325
salads 194, 196
sedentary lifestyles 7, 108, 109,
    150–1
self-awareness 90, 92–123, 117,
    178
    and recording habits 95, 96–9,
        114
    and understanding your day-to-
        day habits 93–5
self-blame 2, 64, 177
self-consciousness 150
self-criticism 273–4
self-esteem, low 384

self-help groups 380
self-kindness 117
self-talk 272–4
selfishness 318–19
sensations 249–50, 251–2
  and the 5-4-3-2-1 grounding
    technique 276
  acceptance 268
  and emotional hunger 102
  getting to know your 260–1
  recording 98, 99, 100–4, **106–7**,
    110–11, 121
  transient nature 264–5
  see also feelings
setbacks 328–38
shame 102, 116–17, 169, 256,
  325
situations, recording 98–100,
  106–7, 108, **110–11**,
  120–2
sleep 258–9
Slimming World 181, 182
SMART principle
  and dealing with other people
    307
  SMART goals 373
  SMART planning 216–21,
    223–4, 227, 242, 247
smartphone apps 332, 372–4
  'habit' 224, 228, 372–3
smoothies 195
snacks
  evening 164
  habits 14, 164
  healthy 137
  sugary 105
social media 8
socialising 144, 236–42
soft drinks 105, 206–7
standing 108, 109
starchy foods **193**, 194, 195
step counters 109, 141, 154–5,
  372

strength training (weight-bearing)
  activity 140
stress
  job 112
  management 121
  recording 121
'stuck' feelings 49, 63–4, 66, 71,
  73, 75–8, 89–90, 114, 116,
  122–3, 216, 238, 242, 253,
  329, 333–8, 362
sugar
  hidden 170
  in soft drinks 206–7
  sugary snacks 105
support 25, 284, 301–2, 332
  lack of 290–5
  psychological 351, 354–7, 377,
    378–9
'surfing the urge' 271–2
surgery, weight loss 348–9, 381
swimming 145

takeaways 6
'talk test' 133
'talking from above' 308–10
television 150–1
temptations 222–3
thinness, ideals of 8, 9
thought errors 64
thoughts 21–2, 58–90
  and 'clearing your head' 305–7
  and emotional eating 265–7
  and hunger 265
  long-term 330–1
  patterns of thinking 24, 58–77
  'permission-giving' 112
  positive 58, 66
  questioning and expanding your
    77–8, 83–4, 362–3
  about setbacks 335–6
  and starting plans 225
  about weight gain 67
  see also automatic thoughts

time issues
  and physical activity 131, 144–5
  and plans 219–20
  and recording information 115
tiredness/fatigue 164, 266
  and dehydration 105
  and overeating 258–9
trade-offs 52–3
treats 232

UK Voluntary Registry of
    Nutritionists (UKVRN) 351

Valium (diazepam) 353
values 40–3, 56, 268–9
vegetables 192–8, **193**
voluntary services 380
vomiting 23

walking 108–9, 131, 138, 140–1,
    149, 153–6, 221, 271
wants, communicating your
    302–3
warm ups 156
weight
  control mechanisms 173–9
  ideal/goal 338–41, 343
  judging others by their 8, 9,
    50–2, 284, 319–22
  maintaining a stable level 234,
    244, 344
  self-consciousness about 150
  see also overweight
weight gain
  after having a baby 253
  after a night out 166–8
  causes of 164
  and children 15, 60, 253
  during a 'slip' 328
  imagining future 44–5, 46–7
  and physical activity 12
  rapid 166–8
  rebound 11, 222–3, 328

resistance to 175–7
and self-awareness 94–5
and soft drinks 206–7
thoughts about 67
weight loss 166
  ambivalent attitudes to 50–1
  automatic thoughts about 67
  costs of 52–3
  and daily life changes 243–6
  and diet types 189, 190–1
  extreme 222–3, 294
  fad theories about 12–13
  getting 'stuck' with 122–3
  imagining future 45–7
  keeping it going 328–57
  knowing where to stop 338–45
  long term 10
  and medication 346–8
  motivations for 17, 24, 31–57,
    341–3
  and muscle mass 130, 176, 177
  permanent 3
  and physical exercise 134–5
  professional help with 345–57
  reasons for 36–43
  slowing down 177–9
  and starting plans 230–1
  stopping 177–9
  and surgery 348–9, 381
  trade-offs 52–3
  working out how much you
    need to lose 25–7
  of yo-yo dieting 2, 3
Weight Watchers 180, 182
weight-bearing activity 140
weight-loss 'experts' 16–18
weight-management groups,
    commercial 187–8
wellbeing 129
whole grains 198–200
willpower 31, 32–3

yo-yo dieting 2, 3, 222–3

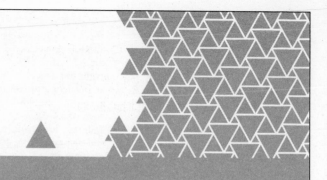

OVERCOMING

Social Anxiety & Shyness

2nd Edition

A self-help guide
using cognitive
behavioural techniques

an
OVERCOMING
publication

READING
WELL

GILLIAN BUTLER

Overcoming Social Anxiety
and Shyness,
2nd Edition

Don't let social anxiety and shyness ruin your life

Everyone feels foolish, embarrassed, judged or criticised at times, but this becomes a problem when it undermines your confidence and prevents you from doing what you want to do. Extreme social anxiety and shyness can be crippling but they are readily treated using Cognitive Behavioural Therapy (CBT).

In this fully revised and updated edition, Dr Gillian Butler provides a practical, easy-to-use self-help course which will be invaluable for those suffering from all degrees of social anxiety.

- Uses real life examples

- Indispensable for those affected by social anxiety or shyness

- Contains a complete self-help programme and worksheets

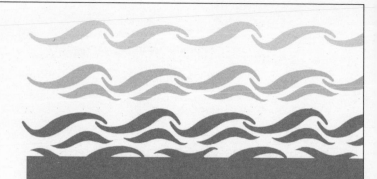

OVERCOMING
Chronic Fatigue
2nd Edition

A self-help guide
using cognitive
behavioural techniques

an
OVERCOMING
publication

MARY BURGESS WITH
TRUDIE CHALDER

READING
WELL   O

Overcoming Chronic Fatigue, 2nd Edition

'Cognitive behaviour therapy appears to be an effective and acceptable treatment for adult out-patients with CFS. Its sufferers deserve . . . to be more aware of the potential of this therapy to bring lasting functional benefit.'

Cochrane R eview

This valuable self-help guide offers ways of improving long-lasting fatigue associated with a range of long-term conditions including chronic fatigue syndrome. Using recognised techniques, cognitive behavioural therapy (CBT) helps to change coping strategies. The approach described helps people break the vicious circle of fatigue and for many results in a reduction in symptoms and disability.

This fully updated new edition provides:

- Guidance on how to improve sleep

- Practical strategies for balancing activity and rest

- Tips on setting and working towards targets that would improve your life

- Step-by-step advice on dealing with blocks to recovery

- Tools for coping with worry and stress

- Ways to challenge unhelpful thoughts

- Suggestions for how partners, relatives and friends can help

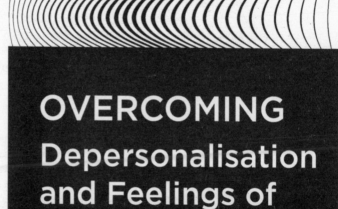

OVERCOMING

Depersonalisation and Feelings of Unreality

2nd Edition

A self-help guide
using cognitive
behavioural techniques

ELAINE HUNTER
DAWN BAKER
EMMA LAWRENCE
ANTHONY DAVID

an
OVERCOMING
publication

O

Overcoming Depersonalisation and Feelings of Unreality, 2nd Edition

'The first of its kind, this self-help book will offer guidance, help and solace to the many sufferers of depersonalization disorder'

Daphne Simeon, Depersonalisation and Dissociation Program, Mount Sinai School of Medicine, New York

Depersonalisation disorder can make you feel detached from life and many people describe feeling 'emotionally numb', unreal or even as if their body doesn't belong to them. It can be a symptom of another problem such as anxiety, depression, post-traumatic stress disorder and, particularly, of panic disorder, or of an illness like epilepsy or migraine. It can also occur in its own right and/or as a side effect of certain drugs.

This self-help book, written by leading experts, will help you to understand what causes depersonalization disorder and what can keep it going, and will introduce you to effective strategies to overcome it:

- Based on clinically proven cognitive behavioural therapy (CBT) techniques

- Clear and accessible step-by-step exercises and tools, including diary-keeping and problem-solving

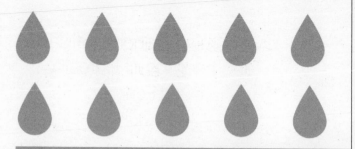

OVERCOMING
Grief

2nd Edition

A self-help guide
using cognitive
behavioural techniques

an
OVERCOMING
publication

O

SUE MORRIS

Overcoming Grief,
2nd edition

Reassuring and helpful strategies to guide you through your grief

Grief is a natural reaction to loss, but in some cases it can be devastating, causing a loss of direction which can impact our relationships and work.

This practical guide will help you to regain a sense of control and offers tried and tested strategies for adjusting to life without your spouse, friend or family member.

Relentless grief can cause a host of physical problems, including difficulties eating, disrupted sleep and becoming over-reliant on alcohol. It can also lead to serious emotional and psychological problems such as depression, anxiety, panic attacks and complicated grief. But techniques from cognitive behavioural therapy (CBT) can help.

This self-help book covers:

- Coping with the unexpected or long-anticipated death of a loved one

- Establishing a routine and tackling avoidance of difficult issues

- Practical concerns such as making decisions and dealing with birthdays and anniversaries

- Returning to work and planning a new future

THE
IMPR⟳VEMENT
ZONE

Looking for life inspiration?

The Improvement Zone has it all, from **expert advice** on how to advance your **career** and boost your **business**, to improving your **relationships**, revitalising your **health** and developing your **mind**.

Whatever your goals, head to our website now.

www.improvementzone.co.uk